# POSITIVELY CAROLINE

# POSITIVELY CAROLINE

## How I beat bulimia for good...
## and found real happiness

Caroline Adams Miller, MAPP

COGENT PUBLISHING NY
IMPRINT OF THE WHITSON GROUP, INC.

Published by Cogent Publishing NY
Imprint of The Whitson Group, Inc.
3 Miller Road, Putnam Valley, NY 10579
www.cogent-publishing.com

The story of my slide into seven years of bulimia and my recovery is true. To protect the anonymity and privacy of others, some names, identifying characteristics and situations have been changed.

Front cover concept and design: DesignSpinner www.designspinner.com
Color photograph on front cover: Scott Robinson
Photograph page 237: Sterling Photography


Manufactured in the United States of America
First Edition

ISBN: 978-0-925776-22-8
1 2 3 4 5 6 7 — 17 16 15 14 13 12

*With gratitude to my brother, Bill Adams,*
*whose support positively changed the course of my life.*

# CONTENTS

# FOREWORD

When you read Caroline Miller's earlier book, *My Name is Caroline*, you are pulled completely into the mind of a young woman struggling with a disease that, at the time of the book's publication in 1988, was rarely acknowledged in public discourse. The immersion into this character is so complete that you feel you know Caroline personally; you celebrate her successes and lament her setbacks as she navigates the rocky road of recovery from bulimia.

In many ways, I shared this experience. At age thirteen, I tore through the pages of *My Name is Caroline* at blazing speed. I turned each page anxiously, utterly engrossed in the story of a woman who was flawed, compelling, and inexplicably relatable. But in another way, my experience was unique. I had been hankering to read this book for a while, but Caroline herself—my mother—had prohibited me from reading the brutally honest memoir of the most difficult time of her life until I was deemed "mature enough."

"The book" was always a part of my life. I remember learning about eating disorders for the first time in my fifth grade "Family Studies" class and being actively bored by the material that I had known for years. I would raise my hand and volunteer the information that my mother had, indeed, suffered from bulimia, and I would receive a stunned silence from my teacher, who would ask if my mother would want me to share something so personal. This always confused me. "It's not, like, a secret," I would counter. "She wrote a *book* about it!"

I proudly showed the girls who came over for play dates our multitude of hardcover and paperback copies of an actual, published book that had a smiling picture of my mother on the cover. I felt famous, and dreamed about one day writing my own book. I begged my mother for years to allow me to read it, because I knew it had been published years before I was born and was terribly curious about her life. Most children do not even consider what their parents were like before they were parents, but I wanted to know everything.

The prohibition was fair: parts of the book are indeed graphic, especially for the eyes of a young girl. I read about my mother binging and purging, drinking and doing drugs, lying and stealing to hide her secret life. But rather than frighten me, the experience of reading *My Name is Caroline* made me feel closer to the woman who cooked my meals and drove my carpools; she was a *person,* not an entity created to serve my needs. When I finished the book, I was content with the knowledge that everything worked out for the captivating woman between the pages. Indeed, I was *living* her future.

But not every reader of *My Name is Caroline* has that same peace of mind. The thousands of letters that flooded my parents' home from women who were previously suffering in silence were a testament to the impact Caroline had on her readers. Since that book ends when my mother was still in her twenties, the question "is long-term recovery possible for women with bulimia?" remains unanswered.

*Positively Caroline* is that answer. Like its predecessor, this book pulls you completely into the mind of Caroline as she deals with her disease in the years after *My Name is Caroline* ends. She becomes even more relatable as she experiences the joys of motherhood, the perils of bankruptcy, the stress of marriage and the dilemma of the work-home balance—all while maintaining her recovery. It is a tremendous story of triumph in the face of personal adversity, but manages to leave this impression without being self-congratulatory. In fact, Caroline is unusually self-aware and consistently willing to work on herself.

Maybe I am a bit biased. Certainly, I love my mother and believe her to be an incredible person. But I love Caroline the character in a way that *any* reader can, and have learned from her experiences through her writing and self-reflection.

*Positively Caroline* is, broadly, a book about dealing with life. It tackles this ambitious task through the specific and personal lens of recovery from bulimia, but its message is universal: know yourself, improve yourself, and love yourself.

SAMANTHA ADAMS MILLER

MARCH 2013

# INTRODUCTION

Exactly twenty-five years ago, I wrote a book called *My Name is Caroline*. In the course of pouring out my story of developing bulimia at 15 in my privileged Washington, D.C. life, I didn't consider the impact my book might have on others… or even on me. I have always needed to write in order to fully experience, understand and process my life, so baring my soul, sharing my worst moments and shame, and chronicling the steady reclamation of my health and happiness was mostly a way to find meaning in my journey and to continue my healing. Even if the book had never found a publisher, I would have been satisfied because writing had given me necessary perspective on my emotional growth.

The book did get published, and my life has not stopped reverberating from the reactions it generated around the world. Not a week has gone by since 1988 that I haven't received a call, email, or letter from someone thanking me for sharing my story. My readers have told me that my honesty gave them hope, and encouraged them to share their own struggles in the course of seeking help. Therapists also tell me that the book served as an introduction to family members who didn't understand a loved one's eating disorder; my story gave them perspective on how to have empathy for the struggle. Many people with eating disorders have used the book as a guide to different approaches on finding their own way to wellness.

In addition to the letters of gratitude and requests for help, I've gotten even more queries about what has happened to me since the book was published. Many ask about Betsy and Annie, who played major roles in my recovery, as well as about my husband, Haywood, who endured years of *petit mal* seizures prior to a *grand mal* seizure when I was just learning how to deal with my eating disorder. "Are you still in recovery? Are Betsy and Annie? Is your husband okay now? Do you have any children?"

I now realize, in hindsight, that I receive these letters because getting into recovery, while very significant, is just the beginning of the struggle that people with eating disorder histories will face. Eating disorder treatment centers in the United States are currently reporting a record-breaking number of middle-aged women streaming in for help—a 42% increase over previous years. Many say that they've been battling eating disorders for decades, never quite finding a way to get into recovery and stay there because of chronic relapse and "addiction switching." Others say that the unending quest for perfection and achievement, coupled with low self-esteem, has caught up to them as their children have left the nest and other life events have shaken them. They are developing eating disorders for the first time at midlife.

Eating disorders are just as prevalent and as dangerous now as they were when I first went public. Eating disorders still have the highest mortality risk of all mental illnesses; 8% of all women are considered to have diagnosable eating disorders. One in five elite female athletes suffers from disordered eating, and one in four college women regularly binge and purge. Body dissatisfaction is prevalent: 80% of women say that they are unhappy with their bodies and have suffered emotionally as a result. Relapse rates are extremely high for people with eating disorders. Indeed, the dieting industry is the only known business to have a 98% relapse rate. There is one very common reason cited for the difficulties in maintaining recovery: although you can abstain from cigarettes, alcohol, drugs and even gambling, food is something you need to touch, smell, prepare, buy and eat throughout each day in order to live. The constant temptation, prompts and opportunities to overeat are too overwhelming for most to withstand slips and full-fledged free-falls back into their old self-destructive ways.

At the close of *My Name is Caroline*, I was 25 and just beginning to think about getting pregnant, which is notoriously challenging for women with eating disorder histories, and I had no role model for how to approach that phase myself. Nor was I prepared for some of the other challenges I would encounter, many of which can trigger relapse. These included coping with morning sickness and weight gain, weathering financial debacles, dealing with post-pregnancy and midlife body changes, being diagnosed with depression and Attention Deficit Hyperactivity Disorder, juggling motherhood and work, treating chaotic family-of-origin issues, and trying to be the best possible role model so that my children would have a chance of avoiding addiction pitfalls.

My main takeaway from the last 25 years is that although *My Name is Caroline* was an important addition to eating disorder recovery literature, *Positively Caroline* could be even more meaningful. In order to truly beat bulimia and all of the emotional minefields that accompany it, I've had to change my definition of recovery, develop a new set of life skills, and work harder than I ever thought possible to become the healthy and happy woman I am today.

So, here's *Positively Caroline*. It is offered in the same spirit as my first book, but is different in many important ways. The first book had the overriding goal of communicating how I went from the emotional and physical bottom of my life to a place where I triumphed over my bulimia. Every chapter was my personal prescription of how to get the Holy Grail: eliminating the eating disorder. No one really knew for sure how to do it back then and I felt it was important to shine a light on my own path in order to try to help others.

Now I want people to see what it means to actually *flourish* in recovery—not just *get there*. Although not all readers will identify with some of the stories I tell, my hope is that the themes of looking for emotional stability post-recovery, developing supportive and meaningful friendships, finding a professional calling, having boundaries with toxic family members, rolling with parenting challenges, finding a balance between fitness and over-exercise, and pursuing my own goals without shortchanging my family will resonate with readers who might benefit from how I managed all of this while staying in recovery.

Another theme of this book is parenting—both the parenting I was given and the parenting I chose for raising my own children. Some of the biggest difficulties I experienced as an adult came from dealing with demons that I wasn't ready to look at when I wrote my first book. Writing *this* book often catapulted me back to dark places that were hard both to re-experience and to put on paper. They are also hard to read.

Most significantly, I share some of what I learned in my extraordinary year in the cutting-edge Master's degree program at the University of Pennsylvania in Applied Positive Psychology—the "science of happiness"—from 2005 to 2006. It was at Penn that I learned that much of what I'd done instinctively to get (and stay) in recovery could be explained through research like Self-Efficacy Theory, Goal Setting Theory, "flow," "positive interventions," the "peak-end" rule, social contagion, the Positivity Ratio, and using "signature strengths." I truly believe that the world of addiction treatment can benefit from Positive Psychology, and that the introduction of many of its principles will make recovery easier and more understandable in its earliest phases.

Overcoming bulimia is the proudest accomplishment of my life. By facing down a disease that I could have easily hidden for several more decades, and then coming out on the other side, I have a perspective and resilience that has served me well in all areas of life and is the touchstone for all of my subsequent growth. As I hit midlife, I am in a physical, emotional and spiritual place that is vastly better than where I was at 20, and I plan to work on making the next few chapters of my life even richer than it is now. I chose the pictures for the book cover as an illustration of where I was as I entered my senior year of high school in 1978 and where I am today. Taken in the same spot on the grounds of Washington's National Cathedral, in the first one I had a full-blown eating disorder, but looked normal to others. In the newer picture, my body is relatively the same, but everything else is completely different—a visible demonstration that illness and recovery don't necessarily have a specific "look," and that true recovery can be invisible to others.

My husband, Haywood, and I will celebrate our 30th anniversary this year. His steadiness at my side has been a large part of my necessary footwork to reach this point. While our marriage isn't perfect and I don't want anyone to think it has been, it's been more honest and strong as a result of our multiple challenges as a couple than it would have been otherwise, and we have created three spectacular children who mean the world to us. I feel blessed that we have "hung in there" together, through everything.

I hope this book hits the right note for those of you who need the messages I've sought to impart. We need more of these types of memoirs so that anyone with an eating disorder will assume that long-term recovery is normal and that there are multiple role models to choose from.

With appreciation and gratitude for everyone who has played a role in a life that I wouldn't ever exchange for anyone else's, I give you this book to finish out the story I began so long ago.

Caroline Adams Miller, MAPP
Bethesda, Maryland
March 2013

# POSITIVELY CAROLINE

# CHAPTER ONE
## EXPECTING THE BEST

I wanted to eat. I wanted hot and spicy chicken wings and I wanted them *now*.

Thoughts of the residential treatment center for eating disorders that my husband and I would open in a few months were temporarily shoved aside. The bulge in my stomach was hungry. Again.

Six years earlier, before my recovery from bulimia, I would have heeded these types of urges by putting on a coat and leaving my comfortable dorm room at Harvard University to go on an all-night binge of ice cream, cookies, and anything else I could get my hands on. Typically, it would end in a dirty, solitary bathroom where I would degrade myself with a long, painful purging session that left me despondent, hopeless and scared.

But here I was now, a pregnant 27-year-old wife in the suburbs of Baltimore, Maryland, a world away from the eight years when I had suffered from bulimia in secret… but feeling the familiar pangs of hunger. Thanks to years of hard work, assistance from a self-help support group, persistence, and therapy, I was now able to make different choices when food beckoned.

"Yes, we are taking applications for various positions," Haywood, my dark-haired, handsome husband said from his desk a few feet away from me. He was dressed in his familiar outfit of jeans, boots and a flannel shirt. Working for ourselves and being home most of the time allowed us this type of freedom and ability to share the day's events, which we both enjoyed.

Word of our treatment center's imminent opening had generated a buzz in the eating disorder field, and we were getting numerous calls every day from prospective patients and therapists who were interested in referring to us or actually enrolling themselves. The Evergreen Renewal Center, our project, sat on 112 acres in Middletown, Maryland, just one hour from where we lived on the outskirts of Baltimore. We were looking forward to giving birth to our first child shortly, and also to a business that could make a difference in many people's lives.

I looked out my office window at the scene before me—trees, horses, pastures, and a few houses that were connected by telephone poles and the lightly paved road at the end of our driveway. I spotted our three horses, Rocky, Trigger, and Donna Buckles, ambling together across the fields, stopping to eat every few steps. I smiled as I gazed at Donna's belly, which was swollen with the imminent birth of her foal. We were *simpatico* in more ways than one. We were both pregnant, hungry, and completely ignorant of the chain of events that would soon turn our worlds upside down.

"Yes, send us your resumé," Haywood continued. "We have already filled some of the top positions, but we are going to be hiring other personnel as we expand."

My husband of six years, who was now also my business partner in starting what would be one of the only residential centers devoted to eating disorder recovery in the country, was handling the business side of our project while I did the marketing. We make a good team in many ways. He has always been able to make me laugh, from the moment we started dating; and our love for each other helped us weather the challenges of my eating disorder, which had spiraled out of control just after we married in June of 1983, one week after my graduation from Harvard.

"I'm bulimic," I'd tearfully admitted to him a few months after we married. It had been a long, miserable day of binging and purging in our apartment while he was at work, and although I'd been dealing with my secret disorder for years by myself, I had finally hit a low enough bottom that I wanted to tell someone, and Haywood was the first person I'd ever trusted enough to reveal my shameful secret. Growing up in the competitive world of private schools and high achievers in Washington, D.C., had left me with the belief that I had to be "the best" to be acceptable. Bulimia definitely wasn't acceptable, so I'd stayed silent, my eating disorder undetected by everyone who knew me during those years.

Haywood had accepted my bulimia admission that night with a mixture of shock, compassion and determination to help me get better. As I began the process of finding the people and resources I needed to help me get on my feet and believe in myself, he stood by me and encouraged me to do whatever I needed to do to win my battle. Without his bottomless support and unconditional love, my journey would have been infinitely harder.

Now we were tackling another major challenge together. As I got better, I'd decided that I wanted to do as much as I could to help other people overcome eating disorders. I wrote a first-person memoir about my life, *My Name is Caroline*, that got an enormous amount of publicity because it was one of the first stories of its kind and the timing was just right. I had also started a non-profit foundation, F.E.E.D., that I ran from my home, distributing free pamphlets about eating disorders and treatment to anyone who wanted that information.

My biggest endeavor, a dream of opening a freestanding residential treatment center in a peaceful setting, had intrigued Haywood so much that he had decided to leave his comfortable law firm job to partner with me in this entrepreneurial adventure. He had chafed at the restrictions and lack of creativity that the legal world offered him, so this venture had appeared to him to be a worthy challenge of his M.B.A., which he had also earned while attending law school.

He had an intensely personal interest in seeing a center like ours open, as well, because nothing like this had been available to me when I needed it most. If we were successful in this undertaking, we both knew that we'd help countless people start their healing process in a serene, safe place.

As Haywood hung up the phone, it was replaced with the insistent ring of another call. This was typical of how we spent our days. We were either going back and forth from the treatment center, making sure the construction was going smoothly and that all of the various permits had been submitted and approved, or we were here in our guesthouse that served as our office, answering calls, taking applications, and giving interviews. Finding out we were expecting a child in the midst of this project had been a surprise, but giving birth to two wonderful labors of love at the same time seemed like a good omen.

❋ ❋ ❋ ❋ ❋ ❋ ❋ ❋

"I'M GOING TO GET SOME LUNCH," I mouthed silently to Haywood, with appropriate hand gestures. He nodded and turned back to the call. I put on my coat and zipped it over my bulbous stomach, eager to stretch my legs and get some fresh air.

The door slammed behind me as I walked out of the guesthouse and headed towards my car. We currently lived in the aptly named town of Boring, Maryland, where we owned a 13-acre "farmette" featuring a main house, the guesthouse I'd just left, and also a pond, three-stall barn, swimming pool, and lots of grass. It was an idyllic spot, and we felt fortunate to have transitioned from the hectic pace of Baltimore city condo living to this "boring" hamlet where the postmistress of our tiny post office still closed up shop to go home for lunch, and where being a good neighbor often meant doing more than just borrowing a cup of sugar. Corralling cows or horses that had escaped a field wasn't uncommon, and we all pitched in. It was a great place to raise a child, we thought, and we looked forward to many happy years in this location.

Our farmette represented more than just a peaceful place to raise a family, though; it was a place where we could retreat from the world and be alone, if desired. Since the publication of my book the previous year, I'd been on a media blitz all over the country, flying from city to city, giving interviews to television and radio shows, as well as appearing on national shows like "The CBS Morning News," "The 700 Club," and CNN's "Sonya Live from L.A."

Although it was fun at times to see my face on the cover of a magazine, or to see excerpts in such widely-read magazines as *Family Circle* and *New Woman*, I also discovered that I was unprepared for the extent of the media scrutiny into my life and my habits. For instance, one reporter from a major newspaper had walked into my kitchen during an interview for a profile and, without permission, had opened the refrigerator to examine its contents.

"I suppose the beer is for Haywood?" she called out, as I sat on my living room couch, too startled to say anything other than a weak "Yes."

On other occasions, I'd gone shopping at the grocery store and noticed people surreptitiously looking into my cart to see if I was buying the binge foods I'd confessed to in the book, like ice cream. And at my support group meetings, where I'd gotten comfort and guidance for four anonymous years, people had begun arriving at the meetings with copies of my book in their hands, hoping that I would sign them or work with them privately as a sponsor. Although I'd known, on some level, that I'd opened myself up to this kind of scrutiny through my candor, it still felt overly intrusive at times, and I wasn't sure how to handle it well.

The tens of thousands of letters that I received from people all over the world weighed most heavily on me, and I took great care to respond to each one. It wasn't uncommon to receive a thick ten-page letter, filled with photographs, that told someone's private story about her (a small percentage of the letters were from men) eating disorder and her unsuccessful attempts to address it. Many of the letters said something like, "After reading your book, I knew that you would understand my problem, and you're the first person I've ever contacted to ask for help. Please write back soon."

Writing a personal note to each person, along with some ideas about what they could do to work towards recovery was important, but time-consuming, and I took the responsibility seriously. Some days I did nothing but write letter after letter, increasingly aware of the impact that my book had had on many lives, and awed by the power that was generated when people suddenly felt hopeful.

The publicity I received was also a big plus for the treatment center. We were able to attract top-notch investors and bankers because they could see how easy it would be to market the facility if I stayed in the news and interest remained high in stories about eating disorder recovery. While there was no way to prove that I had any kind of magic touch, and I never thought or held out the promise that I had all of the answers, it didn't stop people from begging for spots at our center the moment it opened, and many people wanted to send $5,000 deposits just to ensure that they would be admitted first.

One of the biggest endorsements we received was that of our primary investor, Standard Healthtrust, a leader in the fields of inpatient treatment centers, assisted living and retirement homes in the United States. They liked our youth, enthusiasm, business plan, and knowledge of eating disorders, and they wanted to have a stake in this market, which they felt was sure to grow.

Standard's blessing had helped us get favorable bank loans, which Haywood and I had personally guaranteed. At the time, this hadn't seemed like a huge risk because of Standard's reputation, so we'd sat in bank offices for one entire day, signing piles of documents, which assured the center's purchase and also provided us with several months of operating income.

Although Haywood and I had already demonstrated our personal commitment to this venture by raising $120,000 from family and friends, and liquidating all of the stock we had been given as wedding gifts, we had needed Standard's investment and the banks to move ahead with the purchase of the 112-acre estate in Middletown, MD which we then renovated and brought up to hospital code specifications. We had also conducted a national search for a director, and had hired a woman whose experience running numerous for-profit treatment centers made her an outstanding candidate for Renewal's first few years. We gave her an employment contract, and she relocated from Oregon to join us in the months preceding the center's opening.

We had also brought on board a respected psychiatrist in the Washington, D.C. area, who had extensive knowledge of the eating disorder field, to be our medical director. He developed a protocol for treatment that was 12-step based, but also featured many new modalities, such as art and cooking therapy, that we believed would help our clients overcome their fears of food and learn how to express their feelings in safe ways.

To be as current as possible in the operation of successful treatment centers, I had also put myself through a "Professional in Residence" program at the Betty Ford Center in Rancho Mirage, California. Employees there were generous in sharing their staffing and operation guidelines with us, which provided a helpful template for our program. Haywood and I had also toured and stayed at a number of substance abuse treatment centers up and down the east coast, where the directors encouraged us in our mission and said they planned to send us eating disorder sufferers who needed the specialized care they couldn't provide.

As a result, Haywood and I felt like we'd done everything we could to make our venture a winner. We had tackled challenging zoning issues and public hearings in Middletown, and had won against many odds. We had also searched the country for the best people we could find and had sifted through dozens of resumés to hire our key people. When we went to bed at night, we felt confident that we hadn't overlooked any detail in the planning or hiring phases.

If the timing was right, I'd have my child in May and the center would open in September.

Life was good and the future looked bright. Or so I thought.

## CHAPTER TWO
## MY NEON SIGN

I squeezed into my small red Escort to drive to the nearest grocery store. My current bible, *What to Expect When You're Expecting,* said that the seventh month was critical for brain development, so I wasn't shy about eating whenever I was hungry. This was a real shift for me, as was getting in and out of a grocery store without incident. These small changes in my thinking and behavior might seem like miniscule triumphs to someone else, but to me they were all part of the proof that my bulimia recovery was solid and deepening.

It had been six years since I'd walked into the Baltimore support group for compulsive eaters, at which time I was binging and purging multiple times every day, taking dozens of laxatives, and compulsively exercising to burn off extra calories. Shopping for groceries at that time had been a chaotic and unpredictable experience. On some days, I could walk in, buy healthy foods for myself and Haywood, and return home masquerading as a normal person, eating reasonable portions for the rest of the day.

On many other occasions, though, grocery shopping was simply an extended binge session. I'd see a food I wanted, like oatmeal cream pies, and it would trigger the thought that I had to deprive myself of all desserts because I was too heavy. Even though outside observers probably wouldn't agree with my description of myself, I'd thought of myself as "too heavy" ever since my father told a waitress at a restaurant (I was eight): "The vanilla milkshake goes to the heavy one." There had rarely been a period since then

10

that I'd liked myself or my body, and my bulimia had found an easy victim at the age of 15 when some friends had told me that binging and purging was a simple way to stay thin.

Now, with over four years of recovery under my belt, grocery shopping was not the ordeal it used to be. Once, it had been impossible to enter a store without feeling my heart start to pound and fear claw at my insides, but recovery had allowed me to conquer those panicky sensations. Small goals, therapy, and recovering role models—some of whom had been kind enough to walk beside me through the aisles of temptation—had taught me that food shopping didn't have to be the sad and lonely foray it had once been.

Another shift for me had been that pregnancy had widened the circle of foods I'd become familiar with, and that I'd defined as my "safe foods." Prompted by the immediate onset of severe morning sickness, I'd had to change my diet to simple foods—if any on some days—and to confront the constant, all-day nausea without careening back into an easy solution of purging whenever I felt sick. As the morning sickness wore off after three months, I craved heavier and spicier foods. I trusted myself enough to add them gradually to my diet, and stayed in close touch with my friends from my eating disorder support group. I always had people who could hold me accountable, if I needed it.

In fact, I'd reveled in the freedom of my pregnancy clothes, because there was no silent judgment of a belt or a tight waistband if I felt too full. I didn't worry much about whether I'd overeaten, either, because I managed to get a few miles of walking in every morning, and the fit of the rings on my fingers never seemed to change, regardless of how large my stomach got. I also didn't feel drawn to eat the forbidden foods I had once denied myself with the excuse that I could "eat for two;" I just ate more of the foods I craved and that were good for me, and I trusted that everything would turn out well.

I TURNED ONTO the connector road that would take me from Boring to the grocery store fifteen minutes away. As my stomach lurched and the baby did a series of somersaults, I felt an enormous sense of gratitude that I'd been able to get pregnant at all. Many women with eating disorder histories can't perform this basic function because their hormonal levels have been in constant flux for years, their weight is too low for menstruation, and they are under so much stress that their systems don't function correctly.

Another one of my secrets during my eight years of bulimia: I'd never had a single menstrual period, right through my college graduation in 1983. When I was in seventh grade, the most popular book among my friends had been *Are You There God? It's Me, Margaret*, by Judy Blume, which beautifully detailed the longing of every young girl to make the transition from girl to woman with that momentous bloody event, and the jealousy that many pre-teen girls experienced when their friends became "women" before they did.

Like everyone else I'd read the book, but unlike everyone around me, I'd never gotten my period. I'd lied about it out of embarrassment, carrying Tampax with me wherever I went, hoping that it would make me look normal. When people complained about their monthly aches and pains, I clucked sympathetically, acting like I knew exactly what they were talking about, even though I was clueless, and my parents and doctors never thought to ask me if I was having a period at all.

At Harvard, I was part of the first study done on athletes and menstruation, so I'd regularly trooped to the Harvard Center for Population Studies with my swimming teammates and filled out extensive questionnaires about my food, sleep, menstruation and exercise habits throughout my freshman year. Because our data was confidential, I was honest about my unusual physical condition. I hoped that the study results would somehow help me understand my obvious deficiency, which I suspected was related somehow to my crazy eating.

Years later, when these results were published, they laid the groundwork for the well-known "Female Triad" of athletic side-effects: eating disorders, loss of menstruation, and loss of bone density. Although I didn't know it at the time, I was typical of most athletes with eating disorders, but in the early 1980s, this was still unknown data that I couldn't draw upon to help me seek help, so I'd just stayed isolated in my lonely bubble.

After I got married in 1983, though, an amazing thing happened, probably because I felt safe and happy to be with a man who truly loved me, I began to enjoy a life without exams, swimming, and other stresses. Despite the fact that I was still bulimic, my period started with a vengeance in the summer after our wedding, and it mimicked all of the vagaries of a teenager's puberty. Sometimes I got it twice a month and sometimes I got it every few months. Sometimes it was heavy and sometimes it was light. As I entered recovery in early 1984 and overcame my bulimia, my period became more regular. This was another one of the small but significant signs that I was becoming healthier and more normal by the day, and that I was on the right recovery road.

As positive as this development was, though, Haywood and I ran into trouble when we decided to start a family when I was twenty-five. We'd been married for four years, had dated for two years prior to that, I was in recovery, and we wanted to be young parents. My period had been more and more consistent at this point, and the doctor had cleared me to start trying to get pregnant, which we did.

Like many twenty-somethings who are not using birth control, we figured that we'd hit pay dirt within a month or so, but after more than a year of fruitless efforts, we began to wonder if my body had been permanently damaged by my years of purging and delayed menarche. More and more research was coming out about the numerous physical side-effects of bulimia at that time, such as vision change, eroded teeth, electrolyte imbalances and even goiters, so I read as much as possible about what might be contributing to my inability to get pregnant.

One specific fact stood out to me: as many as 60% or more of women in infertility clinics had eating disorder histories. My heart sank when I read this. Had I unknowingly given up my ability to have children when I'd decided that being thin at any cost was my primary goal?

Haywood and I sat down at that point and discussed our options. He was a kid at heart, and an extremely playful man with an easy laugh, so the idea of possibly not having children was particularly hard for him. I felt a terrible sense of shame about the fact that my body was undoubtedly the problem with our fertility challenges, but I took some small comfort in the fact that I was at least in recovery, and that any child we might bring into our family in a different way would have a healthy, happy mom. It was at that point that we decided that we ought to investigate adoption. We started to talk to a few people we knew who had adopted Chinese girls, and who were all delighted with their decisions.

This all occurred just as the hubbub around my book was dying down, and I felt ready to face whatever the future would bring. But my plans were thrown into disarray after I had a dream that was so unusual in its content and message that I was moved to record it in my diary:

*August 15, 1988*

*Last night I had the most incredible dream. The statue of the Virgin Mary in our neighbor's garden was enveloped in an electric blue glow that I've never seen anywhere before. It was unspeakably beautiful. This color was radiating some type of vibrant energy and moving at a lightning-fast pace, like the double-helix DNA patterns I studied in 8th grade science class. I stared at it for a short time or a long time—I don't remember. All I know is that I was mesmerized by the blue hue and the way it was pulsing in and around the statue like a neon sign. No words were spoken, nor did the Virgin Mary gesture in an attempt to communicate with me. But when I woke up, I knew beyond a shadow of a doubt that she had somehow told me I was pregnant.*

Later that afternoon, with shaking hands, I watched as the pregnancy test stick finally, unquestionably, told me that I was going to be a mother.

\* \* \* \* \* \* \* \*

ONE OF THE MOST healing parts of my recovery from bulimia was my gradual adoption of a belief in a Higher Power, which was encouraged in the tenets of my self-help group in Baltimore. As I'd sunk deeper and deeper into my disorder throughout my teen years, I had been attending a private Episcopal girls' school that was affiliated with Washington's National Cathedral, a breathtaking and awe-inspiring building that drew visitors from all over the world, and where I had married Haywood in a flourish of pomp and ceremony in June 1983.

Despite this omnipresent religious setting for nine years of schooling, though, I had never felt any relationship with a force that I could call "God," and I hadn't sensed a loving presence around me as the bulimia overtook my life, either. It also didn't help that I'd always felt like a stray dog who didn't belong anywhere. My family never attended worship services, and none of us had been baptized as babies, so the idea of a spiritual home was completely alien to me. Consequently, I had no soft place to fall when external comforts and security were stripped away.

My Higher Power took shape as I settled into my self-help group because I couldn't explain the transformative power of trust and love I felt without evoking a spiritual explanation. As I gradually healed, I began to see "coincidences" of positive events after I prayed for help or relied on my intuition to guide me to do the "right thing." These led me to believe that there was a loving God who wanted me to get well, and who was sending signs—like my dream about being pregnant—to let me know that my life was on the right track.

In fact, the dream with the dazzling blue lights pulsing around the Virgin Mary resulted in my adoption of an internal barometer that became my go-to signal to move forward. Whenever I needed affirmation or approval of a decision, I would either see a neon sign flashing "Right Way!" in my brain or I wouldn't. It wasn't your normal connection with God, but it worked for me. Consequently I never stopped paying attention to the tiny miracles from the Universe that I saw all around me when I chose to stop, listen and look for God's presence.

The dream about the Virgin Mary statue was, to me, one of those tiny miracles. I interpreted it as a sign from God that despite my years of body loathing and self-abuse, I would be rewarded for my dedication to overcoming bulimia with the blessing of a child. Could life possibly get any better?

# CHAPTER THREE
## HOT AND SPICY

I parked at the grocery store and locked my car. Safely inside the store, I headed for the frozen foods aisle. Although I'd never liked spicy foods before this pregnancy, I'd craved nothing but that since the moment the morning sickness wore off. Sausages, tacos, salsa, and other tangy foods were my new friends. But these wings were special. They satisfied me and the hungry baby inside me in ways that nothing else did.

I grabbed a few packages and headed for the checkout line. "Back again?" the express lane clerk laughed knowingly.

"*He* needs them," I replied.

"It's a he?" she pointed at my striped bulge. "For sure?"

"Just a guess," I said with a smile. "See you tomorrow." I waved and headed back out to the car.

Although I didn't know for certain that I was going to have a son, another strange visionary dream several weeks earlier had led me to think I would. Similar to the one featuring the Virgin Mary, this dream had had a "bigger-than-life" aura to it, and had felt like a special delivery message from the big guy upstairs.

"I'm coming to stay with you," a young boy said as he stretched out his hand to me. I stared at the small child, but didn't reply. He was exquisite: luminous blue eyes, and an innocent face wreathed in white-blond, curly hair. He looked to be about two years old.

I don't remember if we grasped hands or not, but it didn't matter.

When I woke up, I shook Haywood and said, "We're going to have a boy! He's going to have blue eyes and blond curls! He's beautiful! I just met him!"

Haywood, who had learned that nothing was too outlandish when it came to my nocturnal visions, had simply grunted and mumbled, "That's great."

These thoughts occupied my mind during my drive back home to Boring. Although I still wasn't sure how to describe my belief system, I knew beyond a shadow of a doubt that my decision to seek help and stop living a lie had ushered in so many positive "coincidences," kind people, and blessed outcomes that I'd be foolish to ignore the intuition that told me that God was trying to get my attention. But whatever it was, I felt infinitely grateful that my life now appeared to be on track, and I was about to have a child.

\* \* \* \* \* \* \* \*

BACK AT HOME, I met Haywood in the kitchen.

"How are you feeling?" he asked, reaching out to touch my stomach. He felt a responsive thump back and smiled. "When is your next doctor's appointment? Are you gaining enough weight?"

Actually, I didn't know the answer to that last question, but I was entrusting my doctor and his staff to know what was best. From the moment I'd found out I was pregnant, I'd made the choice *not* to monitor my weight gain because I knew the number on the scale could trigger a binge—or at least negative thoughts. I'd focused mostly on widening my circle of foods and becoming comfortable with eating slightly bigger portions. I had come up with a plan, which I explained to my new OB/GYN and his staff at my first visit.

In the office, the nurse had taken my medical history and blood pressure, and then pointed to the scale.

"Time to weigh you," she announced. I felt the familiar lurch in my stomach about being judged by numbers that had never been acceptable to me or anyone else. In fact, I still remembered the night in high school when my parents had brought a scale down to the kitchen and had told me that they wanted to see how much I weighed. I was too fat and they had let me know it in ugly, personal language. Being on the scale and seeing numbers was something I never wanted to do again, if I could help it, so I quickly made a proposal to the nurse about how to handle it.

"I'll get on," I said, "but we need to have an agreement first. Whenever I have to be weighed, I'll turn my back and plug my ears, because I'll know exactly how much I weigh when I hear the bars sliding a certain distance and then stopping." I wish that fact weren't true, but it was. I was so highly sensitized to this torturous process that every detail of moving metal bars on a scale activated my antennae.

The nurse looked at me as though I was crazy, but at least she was listening. I continued.

"You can weigh me under those conditions, but I don't want you to write down the number in front of me or tell me what it is. And at each visit, I only want to be told if I've gained *enough* weight for a healthy pregnancy. That's it."

The nurse paused and said, "Just a minute." She left with a puzzled look on her face and returned with my doctor. He spoke first.

"Caroline, can you tell me a little bit about this, um, request? We need to understand why you are so afraid of knowing your actual weight." He was probably wondering what kind of nut I really was. I gathered my courage.

"I know this sounds strange, but I'm in my fourth year of recovery from bulimia, and this is my first child. I know I have to gain weight, but part of my healing has been not weighing myself or knowing the numbers. I would rather not focus on those things while I'm trying to have a healthy pregnancy. I don't know if it would be a trigger, but I'd rather not find out. So I'd like to just get on the scale backwards, plug my ears, and then you can just record and track my weight yourselves without telling me the number. Okay?" My bookish doctor, who had probably never had anyone quite like me in his practice, thought for a moment, and then nodded.

"Fine with me," was his surprising reply. "Actually," he added, "I think I might have some women like you in my practice already. Maybe we shouldn't tell them what they weigh, either. What do you think?"

Delighted to be consulted as if I were a professional peer, I answered, "Well, do you ask them if they have ever had an eating disorder?"

"No. Why would we?"

"Because of people like me. Even someone who doesn't have a full-fledged eating disorder can get caught up in the fear of weight gain and people commenting on the size of their body. Watching the scale and knowing the numbers might be harder for some patients than you or they realize. So why not offer an option, or just ask if someone has a history that might lend itself to this type of support?"

Again, he pondered my words. "I think that's a great idea." Then he turned to the nurse. "Just put a big sticker on the front of Mrs. Miller's chart saying that this patient doesn't want to know her weight, and that the weigh-in has to be done in whatever fashion makes her comfortable." He turned back to me. "Does that work for you?"

I nodded enthusiastically. "Perfect. I really appreciate it."

So as a result of my speaking up, I had no idea of the weight gain specifics, but I did know that my baby was plenty big and healthy and my blood pressure was normal. I reminded Haywood that the doctor had agreed to tell me if I wasn't doing well.

"How about the dental work?" he asked reaching for some potato chips and chocolate chip cookies to augment his simple lunch of a ham sandwich. "When's that going to be done?"

I was always amazed when I watched Haywood with food. He simply ate to live, without any agony about whether or not it would make him fat. He still had an athlete's body, a vestige of his days as an All-American lacrosse player in high school and college, but he was not overly zealous in his workout regimen, either. His sheer normalcy around food and fitness was always comforting—if not mystifying—to me.

"I have one more visit," I said. "I need to finish before the baby is born, so I'm almost there."

Regular trips to the dentist had been another consequence of my years of bulimia. Whenever I went, however, I told them all about my history, making sure that they understood that any gum recession or subsequent root canals were probably the result of the acid that repeatedly washed over my teeth for many years. My experience with doctors and dentists was similar; they were always interested in what I had to say and were grateful for my candor because it made treatment easier. They also loved to ask questions to better inform their treatment of other patients with similar problems.

* * * * * * * *

AS MY DUE DATE came and went, I became increasingly lethargic and enormous. Finally, at about 3 a.m. on May 7th, 1989, I woke up in tremendous pain. It was time. The baby wanted out.

Naively, I'd anticipated that my lifelong athletic pursuits would make my delivery just like another long workout, with some interval training thrown in, but this was a new and exquisite sensation that I'd never felt before. The pregnancy books definitely hadn't explained it honestly, either. Suddenly every woman in history who had ever given birth was now my hero.

Nine hours later, including lots of moaning and the blessed intervention of an epidural shot to ease my pain, a nurse came in to check my progress as I calmly leafed through the newspaper and observed the contractions on the monitor above me.

"Wow, that's a big one!" Haywood said as he saw the sharp peaks on the screen, indicating that I was in strong labor. "You don't feel any of it?"

I shook my head and was about to praise the wonders of modern medicine when the nurse scurried out to get the doctor, who quickly burst into my room and announced, "It's time to have a baby!" Apparently, the nurse had seen the baby's head crowning when she'd checked the extent of my dilation, and was concerned that we wouldn't make it into the delivery room in time, so they flew me down the hallway, with Haywood in hot pursuit.

21

After a few pushes, I felt something the size of a football shoot straight out of me, and my stomach suddenly deflated like a bad soufflé.

"He's so heavy!" I heard a nurse say in wonderment, as a baby's screams filled the room. That was the moment at which I learned I'd had a boy, and a big one at that.

I looked over in tired, but profound, awe. Haywood was leaning against the wall, white as a board, with a camera in his hand. I saw him try to take a picture, but he put the camera down. Instead, he moved toward the sink where our son was being washed and counted the number of fingers and toes, which he told me later was all he could think to do.

Then my gorgeous, ten-pound firstborn was laid on my chest. He looked right up at me, and his blue eyes met mine. It was a moment of instant recognition: he was unmistakably the child I'd seen in my dream.

* * * * * * * *

THAT FIRST NIGHT I refused to allow my son to be taken to the nursery with the other infants, so he slept right at my bedside so that I could scoop him up and nurse him the moment he moved or cried. I had never experienced such feelings of completeness and exquisite happiness. I couldn't stop smiling or looking at him, scrutinizing every perfect feature, from his fair eyebrows to his little fingernails. It was amazing to me that my body had produced this miracle. Along with that sensation, I felt a fierce, all-encompassing love throughout my being that I'd never felt before. I also knew that as much as I'd had to love myself and fight for myself to recover and even have a body that worked normally, I'd fight even harder if this child were ever in danger.

During the second day at the hospital, flowers, cards, and calls streamed in, all with warm wishes and congratulations. I took my first shower and ran my hands over my body, which had felt so alien for so many months. I looked down and could see my feet, which I hadn't been able to do for quite a while.

Daddy Haywood came to visit at the end of the second day, but left within two hours to handle some "important" calls about Renewal. Although he was ecstatic about the birth of our son, something seemed to be bothering him. I brushed it off, thinking it might be just another stray zoning or permit issue we needed to satisfy. These problems had been a bit like the game "Whack A Mole," because every time we'd think we were done, another problem would arise.

The following day dawned bright and warm, and I dressed excitedly because I'd be introducing our baby to the home where I knew he'd spend many happy years. I nursed him while waiting for my husband's arrival. When I heard Haywood's familiar step coming down the hall, I smiled in anticipation.

Haywood walked in with a look I'd never seen before. The smile disappeared from my face and the temperature of the room seemed to drop.

"Caroline," he said, fixing me with a stare and then glancing at our newborn. "Yesterday, Standard Healthtrust decided to pull out of our project. They said it was for private reasons and not because they don't believe in our center. But I've also been talking to the banks. They might not want to participate without Standard involved, which may be a hurdle that we can't get past in time for the scheduled opening in the fall."

My body went into shock and my brain suddenly felt numb. After more than two years of great news and forward progress on every front, this was a major, unexpected blow.

"What does this mean for us?" I asked in confusion, thinking that I might have misheard him somehow, and that I'd return in a moment to the blissful afterglow of childbirth.

"Well," he answered carefully, "if the banks pull out and we can't find a replacement, we are responsible for all of the loans on the center, and we obviously don't have that kind of money." Indeed, everything we had ever possessed had gone toward making our dream come true.

"We may have just lost everything we own," Haywood said.

I looked at my son, back at my husband, and closed my eyes. This couldn't be.

A tug on my breast jolted me back to reality. I looked down at my baby, trying not to cry. Talk about bad timing. At least he was oblivious. My fingers traced the contours of his fuzzy head, his tiny ear, his soft back. He nursed contentedly, eyes shut tight. The room was silent, except for his gulping noises. How could something so beautiful be juxtaposed with something so awful?

"You know C," said Haywood, using his nickname for me, "we'll be okay. I'm just not sure how. I'm so sorry this is happening. I know you want to enjoy the baby right now." He gently reached out to caress our child.

Finally I looked up at him. He had done the best he could, and so had I. Maybe we'd find a new backer if we got out of the hospital quickly and made a bunch of phone calls.

As our new family of three left the hospital, we knew we had a fresh set of battles ahead of us and that our lives were going to be different forever.

Little did we know *how* different.

# CHAPTER FOUR
## ONE DAY AT A TIME

"Uh uh uh..." the baby monitor in my office came alive with the sounds of Haywood waking up from his afternoon nap. Grateful for any interruption, I began a slow jog from my office on the far end of the 7,000-square-foot estate, through a common area, two offices, the kitchen, a long hallway, and up a sweeping staircase to my son's bedroom. As I got closer, I could hear happy chatter. I smiled in spite of how I was feeling.

A huge, blond, toothless boy squirmed to see me over the bunting in his crib. His expansive grin made me forget for a moment that we were squatting in a house that wasn't ours while our professional lives were unraveling. In an unexpectedly dire turn of events, we'd had to abruptly sell our Boring farm and move into the treatment center to try to salvage our dream, so that was now our cavernous home.

I picked him up and grimaced. Gigantic from the start, Haywood was getting bigger by the day and pushing the limits on the percentile charts for height and weight, possibly because he was sucking down prodigious quantities of formula. Although I'd wanted to nurse my baby for as long as possible, the packing, moving, and stress of leaving our home had disrupted my breastfeeding schedule and forced me to wean him long before I had wanted to. The suddenness of this change had also caused my hormones to drop precipitously, amplifying my already bleak mood.

On top of that, instead of spending Haywood's first few weeks enjoying his every movement and breath, my days had primarily revolved around looking for a financial savior and trying to salvage the company while caring for my baby with worried and divided attention. In fact, less than two weeks after giving birth, I'd gone against doctor's orders and made a business trip to Boston. Although I knew it was unwise to do so, a large investment group that had the potential to save Renewal had requested a promising meeting, and I'd felt that I had no choice but to grit my teeth and go with my newborn in my arms.

One exception to this challenging time and what it took away from the joy of new motherhood occurred on the Sunday after I gave birth to Haywood, which happened to be Mother's Day. As I'd reveled in the joy of holding and nursing my newborn in an Adirondack chair overlooking our shimmering pond in Boring, I realized for the first time how meaningful that holiday would always be for me going forward, and how grateful I was for the privilege of becoming a mother.

While I rubbed Haywood's soft head and gently caressed his delicate fingers and toes, I vowed that his father and I would find a way to give him more security in the future. I also silently promised that this current chaos would not be the environment he would live in forever.

Despite our financially dire circumstances, I hadn't lost sight of the fact that having a healthy baby and nursing him successfully were two more pieces of evidence that my recovery was strong and that I'd worked extremely hard to change the behaviors that had once kept me from having a menstrual period or even knowing how to feed myself. Weathering the nausea of morning sickness, broadening the circle of foods that I could eat without fear, even gaining weight without obsessively monitoring the numbers had all been unexpected positive byproducts of getting pregnant.

Whereas I had once judged my recovery by how long it had been since I'd binged and purged, my definition of successful recovery now also included staying on track regardless of the physical changes to my body, and developing a far more flexible plan of food choices than I'd once had in my early "abstinence" days.

My pregnancy had also been a beacon of hope for many of the women in my eating disorder support group, who had thrown me a surprise baby shower in my second trimester. Because so many of them still struggled with similar issues of menstrual irregularities, and a fear that the weight gain of pregnancy would be too difficult to handle without sliding backwards, I'd been happy to share my various solutions to these challenges, such as getting weighed backwards at the doctor's office.

With Renewal's challenges, it felt especially awkward that this period coincided with being named *Self* magazine's "Person of the Month" for my book and contributions to the eating disorder field. I wore a false smile as I posed for the photographer, perched on our pink couch in the bay window overlooking our pond. Only those closest to us knew that our days were anything but happy, and that we were tearfully giving away our horses to good homes, selling a property at a loss that we had hoped would be our home for many more years, and packing up our belongings to move to a town where we knew no one except people who had been involved in buying, staffing and renovating the property for the treatment center. All family, friends and other familiar situations would soon be more than an hour away from a bucolic town close to Antietam, the site of the bloodiest battle of the Civil War. Perhaps it was fitting that our dream might die so close to this historic, but tragic, spot.

It wasn't just our personal situation that kept me awake at night. It looked like in addition to losing all of the money we'd invested, we were also going to lose the money of the family members and friends who had so generously backed our dream in exchange for now worthless stock certificates. Disappointing them and telling them that their trust in us had been misplaced would be one of the hardest and most embarrassing tasks of my life. Whereas my bulimia had mostly hurt myself, this grand failure was going to hurt a lot of people in ways that pierced me to the core.

I LIFTED HAYWOOD out of his crib and laid him down on the changing table. No matter how many diapers I'd changed since he was born, I loved this ritual because it allowed us to connect in wonderfully unexpected ways. I was rubbing his belly and cooing when my husband burst through the door to join us.

"How's my boy?" Haywood boomed. "There's my Little Man!"

Big blue eyes gazed up in gleeful recognition and fat legs wriggled happily.

"He's going to be a football player. Just look at his size," Haywood chortled.

I was already accustomed to hearing Haywood discuss his son's possible future athletic exploits, and all of the sports that he would play as he grew up and entered manhood. Although I knew Haywood would have been delighted with either a son or a daughter, anticipating the possible athletic path of a son clearly gave him something to be excited about, and that he was familiar with, at a time when we both needed something to look forward to and cheer us up.

"Any hopeful news about Renewal?" I knew it was a long shot, but still found myself feeling naively optimistic at times.

"I don't think so, C."

I finished changing Haywood's diaper and handed him to his father. No wonder he was a happy baby; he had both parents around him all the time, and regardless of what was going on, we managed to always meet his needs. He had never been left alone with anyone but his mom or his dad, so he was pretty securely attached to us, burbling contentedly most of the time and providing our lives with some of their only bright spots.

Haywood hefted his son over his shoulder and walked into our bedroom through the shared bathroom. He laid Haywood down on the bed and began to play the peek-a-boo game they both loved.

Our son shrieked in delight at his dad's game. Thank goodness he was too young to understand that his parents, who had desperately wanted him to be born and who doted on his every move, were now unsure of how they would make ends meet or even where we would raise him. Although we still owned our small condominium in Baltimore, it was rented out for another year at a rate that barely covered its mortgage, and we had no other properties, assets or money to our name.

We were close to penniless except for the condo. On top of investing everything in Renewal, we'd sold our farmette at no profit and we had no jobs and no income, except for the remaining months of operating expenses that would have to sustain us until it ran out. Without Standard Healthtrust, or someone to replace them, we were headed for a Chapter 7 bankruptcy filing, and would face many years of repaying several hundred thousand dollars of loans to our creditors, unless we wanted to declare personal bankruptcy through Chapter 11 and completely walk away from all debt. That, however, wasn't something Haywood or I had ever discussed, nor did I think we were capable of personally flying that white flag of defeat and having everyone else shoulder the burden of our misfortune.

In less than six months, I'd gone from being realistically optimistic about my future to this current miserable scenario where pessimism ruled. It was incredibly hard to wrap my brain around the speed and severity of our downfall.

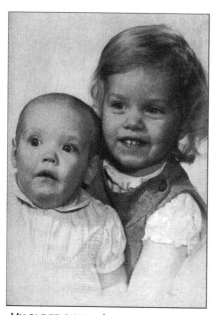

My older sister, Lizzie, holds on to me in an early portrait.

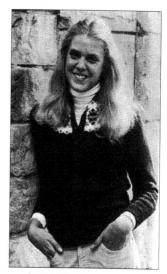

Although the senior picture in my high school yearbook showed a seemingly happy, healthy young woman, I was really hiding my bulimia from the world, which I'd already been practicing for over two years.

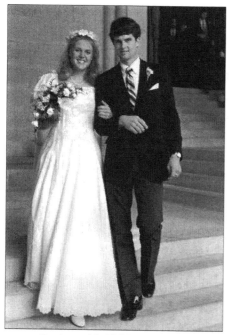

On June 18, 1983 I married H. Haywood Miller, III in an elaborate ceremony at Washington's National Cathedral.

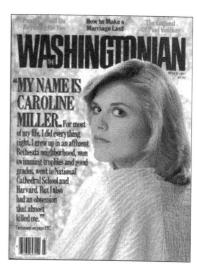

"My Name is Caroline," was excerpted in the Washingtonian Magazine, featuring me on the cover. The following year, the book was published and my entire life turned upside-down.

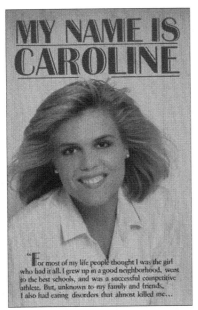

# MY NAME IS CAROLINE

"For most of my life people thought I was the girl who had it all. I grew up in a good neighborhood, went to the best schools, and was a successful competitive athlete. But, unknown to my family and friends, I also had eating disorders that almost killed me…"

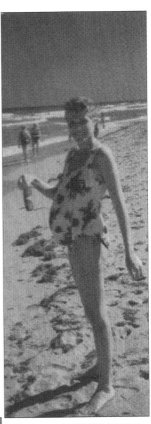

NOT A WEEK HAS GONE BY SINCE PUBLICATION OF "MY NAME IS CAROLINE" IN 1988 THAT I HAVEN'T RECEIVED A CALL, EMAIL, OR LETTER FROM SOMEONE THANKING ME FOR SHARING MY STORY.

DURING MY PREGNANCIES I STOOD ON THE SCALE BACKWARDS AND PLUGGED MY EARS SO THE DOCTORS COULD RECORD AND TRACK MY WEIGHT WITHOUT EVER TELLING ME THE NUMBER.

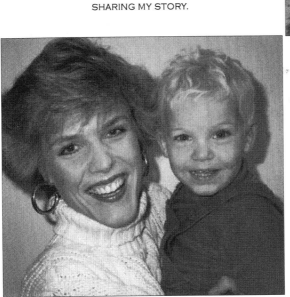

WHEN HAYWOOD WAS AROUND 18 MONTHS OLD, HE LOOKED EXACTLY LIKE THE SMALL CHILD WHO'D COME TO ME IN A DREAM IN 1988 AND TOLD ME I'D GIVE BIRTH TO A BOY.

31

## CHAPTER FIVE
## THIN ISN'T IN

Although it was only four o'clock in the afternoon, I wanted to sleep. I needed to escape my despair over this nightmare. I slouched back into the bathroom and stared into the massive mirror over the matching sinks. My eyes were dark, hollow pits and my usually full face now had cheekbones that jutted out sharply. My hair was lifeless and dull. It occurred to me that I resembled a zombie in a horror movie.

What's more, my body looked surprisingly thin, and it seemed like my pre-pregnancy clothes were even a bit big on me. Because of the seriousness of the numerous other issues I'd needed to pay attention to since Haywood's birth, food hadn't been on my mind much, and it showed. It was suddenly obvious that trying to salvage the treatment center and spending long days and nights tending to an infant had taken their toll on my body, not just my mind.

"Haywood, how do I look to you? Do I look too thin?"

I emerged from the bathroom and turned every which way to ensure that he didn't miss an angle. I even lifted my shirt a bit so he could see what was left of my "pregnancy stomach."

"Yes," he replied without even looking at me. "I'm glad you asked."

I went back into the bathroom to examine myself again. I could see that I looked distinctly thinner than I'd been before I got pregnant. Oddly enough, that realization didn't please me.

As I gazed at myself in the mirror, I reflected on all of the years when

I had wished that I could be effortlessly lithe and slender, and not always hear the words "big," "solid" or "athletic" applied to descriptions of me. My drive to be thin and known as "skinny" like my older sister, Lizzie, or many of the other girls at my prep school, had occupied my thoughts and behavior for too many years, siphoning off precious time and energy that I hadn't devoted to friendships, hobbies or being happy with myself. This obsession had primed me to be the perfect bulimia victim, so when two girls had told me at the age of 15 that they used vomiting to stay thin after overeating, I'd been only too eager to try it, and had quickly gotten hooked.

My weight in recent years of recovery had felt extremely comfortable, but "thin" hadn't been a word used to describe me then either, although it hadn't really bothered me. I had just been happy that my clothes fit from day to day, that my food was stable, and that my energy and zest for life had returned.

"You look healthy," was the phrase that was used most often to describe me, and because my primary goal had been to recover my health, it had seemed like the perfect compliment.

But what I saw in the mirror now was what I'd once wanted long ago—skinniness—and it looked ugly. I was now, finally, thin, and probably even too thin. I was reminded of a phrase I'd read once in a magazine: "Men don't want to make love to a coat rack." I could see why; I looked like a coat rack and there was nothing appealing about it, even to me.

"This was the body I prayed for?" I wondered as I stared at myself. Lord, if only I'd known that reality wasn't as desirable as the fantasy I'd created around it, I might never have had an eating disorder, or spent so many years hating how I looked. That thought, and all that it meant about wasted years, hit me with a sickening thud.

"Do you think I might have a problem?" I asked Haywood, peering around the doorframe and into our bedroom. These bedrooms and the bathroom constituted the "home" that the three of us inhabited when we weren't thousands of square feet away in our offices. Once we were up here at the end of the afternoon, it was hard to motivate ourselves to trudge back down to our cheerless offices and the clanging phones.

"No, but I think you *could* be eating more. I know you're not bulimic because I'm with you all the time, and I would have noticed if you were in the bathroom throwing up, so I'm not worried about that. Have you seen or talked to your sponsor lately?"

That was a good question without a good answer. When I'd entered my self-help fellowship for compulsive eaters in 1984 at my worst bottom, I'd asked several different women to help guide me through creating daily recovery. These people were known as "sponsors," and as I'd gotten better, I'd also become a sponsor for other people. This simple form of honesty and accountability for change made up the backbone of a variety of similar programs for recovery from alcoholism, gambling, and drug abuse, and I'd benefited immensely from this process and the ensuing friendships that had been forged. It had been a rare day that I hadn't talked to one or more people in my program for years, and Haywood's question pinpointed another loss I hadn't been aware of.

Ever since I'd had the baby and moved to Middletown, my life had been nothing but travel, meetings, negotiations, and tending to a newborn. I'd also been hiding our downward spiral from program friends, trying to keep up appearances, prevent the widespread news that our center might not open, and avoid what I was sure would be their pity. I didn't even know if I'd given many of my program friends my new phone number, so it was possible they wouldn't even know how to reach me if they had wanted to.

As I silently contemplated Haywood's question, it also hit me that what I perceived as my shameful failure had led me to isolate myself in Middletown on a lonely estate, separated from everything and everyone who'd ever mattered to me, just as I'd done with my bulimia for many years. Although I'd nurtured my support group friendships and relied upon them during many tough times as I'd gotten well, the success of my book, the intense publicity around it, and the demands of the treatment center had often kept me away from the continuity of the meetings and its wonderful people. They had been as excited about Renewal's potential for positive change as I was, and now I was shutting them out and not letting them see my pain out of sheer embarrassment.

I suddenly realized that I had once had similar feelings of desperation and loneliness around my bulimia, but that being humble enough to reach out and ask for help then, despite my pain, had saved my life. It was now time for me to be humble and reach out for help again, because going through this next phase of life alone was going to be impossible.

* * * * * * * *

WHEN I'D ENTERED my free self-help support group for compulsive eaters in early 1984, I'd instantly found men and women who spoke my language and who all struggled with the common enemy of food, whether they ate too much, starved themselves, or got rid of the calories in a self-destructive way.

Betsy, a tall, attractive blonde, had riveted me at an early meeting with her detailed rendition of going on horrific food-buying sprees, and then vomiting into grocery bags. When she finished her story, with an invigorating account of how she was recovering one day at a time, my life turned upside-down in the best possible way because she was the first person ever to give me hope that my life could get better. I dated the beginning of my recovery to hearing Betsy's unvarnished story and I always credited God with putting me in the right place at the right time to hear her message.

I asked Betsy that night to sponsor me in taking the first few steps of the program, and she graciously talked to me on the phone on countless subsequent occasions when my resolve was shaky, or I needed to simply confess a slip in my eating. Sadly, as my recovery got stronger, hers weakened until she eventually became a fulltime bulimic again, getting fired from multiple jobs because of her well-known and increasingly damaging behavior. In one painful episode, I confronted her upon encountering her jogging near my home, her emaciated frame betraying her condition. Her refusal to accept my offer of help still haunts me, and underscores how important it is to remain vigilant about recovery, and to ask for, and accept, help when necessary. If nothing else, watching her had shown me that getting into recovery was a positive first step, but that staying in recovery was a far more difficult task than even she'd expected.

After that, I'd turned to a very different woman to guide me through my next phase of recovery. Annie was as different from Betsy as she could be. Whereas Betsy was tall, Annie was small. Betsy was an old-line WASP with a blueblood background; Annie was the daughter of Jewish immigrants. Betsy was earthy in her terminology; Annie was proper. Betsy was quick to laugh; Annie was quiet and thoughtful. Despite these many differences, Annie's support was just as instrumental in my recovery as Betsy's guidance had been, and it was she who now got the call that I needed help.

"Annie, it's Caroline," I said the next day on the phone.

"Gosh! Long time, no hear!" she laughed. "Word has it that you left town suddenly... is that true? I haven't seen you at meetings, and I know you have a baby, but I figured I would run into you somewhere, and I haven't. So what's up? Did you actually move?"

I took a deep breath. "Yes, I did move, and it was really abrupt, so I'm sorry I didn't let you know. It was a hard time, and we're not really settled here as it is." I took a few minutes to fill Annie in on Renewal's situation and what it meant for us, asking her to keep my news to herself until I was ready to share it more widely within our group.

"But that's not actually what I called you about," I added, after thanking her for just listening to my story without any judgment or commentary.

"Annie, I need help for something else," I confessed, "and it's a bit strange to even admit this to anyone, given my history."

"What? Did you have a slip with the bulimia and you're too embarrassed to tell anyone because of the book?"

"No," I said, laughing ruefully. "Not that, thank goodness. It's actually the opposite. I think I might actually be too thin right now, and as much as I always wanted to be skinny, I'm just noticing that I may have lost a bit too much weight while breastfeeding and dealing with a lot of professional anxieties.

"I'm not skinny like 'anorexic skinny,'" I hastened to add. "I just think I'm probably about five pounds or so under what I normally am, and Haywood agrees that I might be too thin. It's not horrible, but if it continues like this, I could really get sick."

"What part do you most need help with?" One of the things I love most about Annie and others in the program is that they tend to be fairly unflappable around food topics. It was pretty hard not to find people who had similar stories around food abuse, regardless of the actual details, which was very comforting. If someone had confessed to robbing a bank to pay for a binge at a meeting, I often felt we'd all say, "Thanks for sharing," and then offer our supportive ideas about how to deal with it.

"I guess I need help understanding how to gain weight without going overboard," I answered. "I know I'm not clinically anorexic, because I know I don't have that obsessive desire to eat nothing and exercise all day, and I didn't have a goal to actually lose weight recently. In fact, I definitely eat and I don't even exercise that much these days. But you've said that you were too skinny at times in your recovery, so I thought you'd be the perfect person to ask about how to gain weight in a stable, healthy way."

We talked for a while about how Annie had once used a macrobiotic diet to control her food intake, and how that excessive caution had led her to be anemic, skinny and unhappy.

"My hair even started to fall out," Annie remembered with a rueful laugh, "but I kept saying to myself that I was in recovery, and I wasn't binging and purging, so it was okay."

"What happened to change your mind?" I asked. I was really glad I had made this call to Annie; I was already feeling relieved about my confession and honest desire to get help.

"Bill and I were going to a restaurant for a special night out to plan our wedding," she reminisced. "I was still following a macrobiotic diet and I carried things like salad dressing with me, just in case they didn't have the right things at the restaurant for my eating plan. So that night I opened my purse at the restaurant and the salad dressing was all over the inside of my purse, on my checkbook and everywhere else. It was disgusting and I started to cry, so we left the restaurant and went home. That night I realized that my food plan had become a prison, and that it was so inflexible that it was not only alienating people I loved, it was keeping me from fully enjoying life. Instead of nourishing myself and having a healthy recovery, I was chronically under-eating and being miserable because my food guidelines were so narrow. I was not binging and purging, but I wasn't really living in happy recovery, either."

I was momentarily silent as I contemplated her story. "So what did you do? How did you go about gaining weight without freaking out?"

"The same way I stopped purging—one day at a time. I ate a little bit more of the foods I liked, and I let go of the control around whether or not it was a perfect macrobiotic meal. That simple act of surrendering was what I needed to do to relax into my recovery and slowly put on weight. I did it gradually, and I got rid of a lot of the clothes that were in small sizes so that I was only looking forward to the size I wanted to be. I made myself accountable to a number of people in the program, as well as Bill, to remind me not to undereat or give in to the temptation to be the "perfect" macro-biotic devotee, and that helped me to keep my resolve. It worked. I'm now at a healthy size, I'm not as moody as I was when I was obsessed with my meal plan, and I've redefined recovery to mean that I'm not being so rigid about food that I undernourish myself, instead of just defining recovery as not binging and purging."

Annie had given me a lot to think about. We talked a bit longer, and she offered to drive out to Middletown to spend time with me so that I could show her the treatment center that would probably never open, check my perceptions about my body against her reality, and have a longer conversa-tion about this topic in person. None of my program friends had been out to Middletown to see Renewal because they had all been waiting for the grand opening scheduled for next month, but I wanted to show at least one pro-gram person what Haywood and I had been doing so that I could feel some sense of pride in our journey. No one would ever heal from their eating dis-order here, but maybe it would be the home for me to heal in a different way.

## CHAPTER SIX
## YOU'RE ONLY AS SICK AS YOUR SECRETS

Annie and I settled into the chairs at the table in the area that made up our breakfast nook. Bay windows surrounded us, providing yet another gorgeous vantage point of the vast, verdant backyard. Despite the view, the kitchen was antiseptic and impersonal, and the only sign that this wasn't a hospital facility was the colorful high chair that sat between two long counters, and the gaudy plastic baby pool on the stone patio outside the back door. Even the sinks were industrial-size; they were so huge that I'd bathed my son in them on many occasions. In fact, everything in this room was super-sized and built for a crowd, not a family.

"You are a little bit too thin," Annie opened as we got comfortable, "and I knew you wanted my opinion after seeing you in person."

"Is it really awful? I mean, do I look scrawny?"

I was still perplexed that I'd lost weight without truly realizing that I'd overshot the setpoint that had been so comfortable during my recovery years. Not knowing how much I weighed before I'd gotten pregnant, how much I'd gained during the pregnancy, and how much I weighed now, further complicated the situation because I didn't have any natural method of monitoring myself, other than how I intuitively felt or how my clothes felt. Clearly, simply judging how much to eat based upon my feelings wasn't always accurate, nor were my clothes, which had mostly consisted of stretchy pregnancy outfits in the last year.

"Look, I've known you for a long time, and I saw you at your first meeting when you were still bulimic and your face was swollen and your body was, too. I watched you settle into a healthier, thinner body over the last few years, and you've really looked pretty much the same the entire time. You even looked great while you were pregnant, and I know you were successful at widening your group of safe foods as your cravings changed and you dealt with morning sickness, so you've gone through a lot of changes without going haywire."

Annie's words didn't feel like a judgment or criticism of me or my character, so I welcomed her thoughts. Her demonstrated compassion for me also had deep roots, and her knowledge of who I was and how I appeared to her today were grounded in factual context.

Prior to befriending people like Annie, whom I'd allowed to see deep into my soul, I'd more often felt the sting of criticism from my mother and father, who would tell me that I was unattractive and heavy in high school, or from people who met me during my recovering years, and who mistakenly assumed that my healthy appearance was simply the easy result of inheriting a lanky, athletic build from my parents. After enduring years of these types of inaccurate judgments, asking for and receiving honest feedback about my body was a delicate subject that I only entrusted to a few, carefully selected people.

"Honestly, it's not awful, but your face looks a little bit thin, and so do your arms."

I looked down at my arms, and for the first time saw them as noodles. I'd always been proud of being a strong athlete, but that had taken a backseat since I'd given birth. I didn't see a single muscle. The coat rack analogy came to mind again.

"Anything else?"

"You also look really sad, and that makes you look thinner, too. I've never seen you look like this, and I wish I could make this whole thing better for you in some way. I can't imagine how hard it must be for you to be out here, dealing with this alone. Please reach out to me more often. I had no idea how badly things have worked out for you, and I don't think anyone else does, either." She reached out to put a slender hand on top of mine.

Annie's simple gesture of kindness uncorked my grief. My tears cascaded down my cheeks as I confided all of my financial fears.

Annie let me cry for a while, and then we returned to the topic of my body. "Do you think you've just lost interest in food?" she asked. "When you eat, what do you eat?"

I got up to show Annie the contents of our refrigerators and the walk-in pantry. "I never run out of baby food," I laughed, showing her the dozens of jars of pureed carrots and boxes of oatmeal.

"But I guess I don't have a lot of variety for myself when I eat because it feels like a boring chore to just make a meal. Sometimes I'm just not hungry, so if I'm going by how I feel intuitively, my body isn't giving me the right signals that it needs to be fed regularly."

Annie went back to the refrigerator to inspect its contents. "How about a sandwich? Can you eat a sandwich and fruit for a meal?"

"I hate to make excuses, but you have no idea how often I've wanted to make something like that and I've come in here to find out that we don't have the ingredients. At that point, I don't want to get into the car and drive fifteen minutes to a grocery store, so I just settle for cereal because it's easy and fast. Haywood often eats before he drives home from work, or he picks at whatever we have. I don't even want to be in this kitchen for very long—who would want to be? There isn't a personal touch in here other than the high chair. Everything I look at is just a reminder of the fact that I live in a treatment center that will never open! In fact, I feel like this is a huge hospital and that I've become the main patient."

Annie was quiet as she digested my words.

"Okay, so what I'm hearing is that it's a lot of work to make sure you have the food you want, your mood is preventing you from feeling hungry at times, and you don't even enjoy the surroundings you're eating in. Do you ever go out to a restaurant?"

"Annie, we can't afford it. There is no room in our budget for a restaurant of any kind—even a fast food chain. It's that bad. Really—I'm not exaggerating."

"Okay, okay," she said soothingly, trying to head off another emotional upset. "Caroline, you just need to go back and use all of the tools you used to get into recovery from bulimia. Plan your meals, have the right foods around at all times, connect with healthy people who care about you, and tackle this one day at a time. You can do anything one day at a time. Don't ever forget that."

Her words were simple and profound, as well as accurate. I needed to face my challenge with a plan, accountability and hope, and change these things one day at a time. I felt tension leave my body, replaced by relief that I had a trusted ally at my side for this battle.

I wiped away any remaining tears and looked squarely at Annie. "I'm ready. Will you help me? I really don't want to be this thin, and I never want to be accused of having an eating disorder, because no one who reads my book will believe me if I don't radiate health. If this treatment center doesn't work out, at least my book will continue to spread some positive messages and hope to people who need it."

"Of course I'll help you," Annie said, shutting the refrigerator and sitting down at the table to write out my plan.

"Let's make a list of the foods you like and you can eat without worrying. Then why don't we go to the store and buy them, and come back and stock the place for the next two weeks? If you don't have enough money, I'll pay for it. You just need to get going."

One of the slogans I'd often heard in my program that I loved was, "HALT—Don't get too Hungry, Angry, Lonely or Tired." I'd managed to get hungry, angry, lonely AND tired recently, so it was no wonder that I'd neglected my self-care and my tank was running on empty.

As Annie and I clambered into her small car to make the drive to the grocery store, I experienced the first genuine surges of hope in months that my life would ultimately be okay. I didn't know exactly how that was going to happen, nor did I have any idea when or if we'd ever be completely out of debt, but the little voice that I'd relied upon to help me make wise decisions in recent years now whispered to me, "Don't worry, be happy," as the center faded from the rear view mirror of the car.

I'm glad I didn't know at that moment just how much harder and longer my journey would be. If I'd known, my own journey of recovery from bulimia, and Renewal's struggles to survive, would have looked like a piece of cake.

## CHAPTER SEVEN
## HAPPINESS IS AN INSIDE JOB

The months after my conversation with Annie were spent taking better care of myself and making sure that I regularly nurtured my body in a more loving way. For example, whenever I fed my son, I took note of whether or not I had eaten enough that day too, and I double-checked that we always had enough supplies in the refrigerator to get through the week. Instead of eating intuitively, I also ate more than I wanted to on occasion, simply because I knew that my hunger cues weren't the right barometer of what I really needed during times of extreme stress.

Although my weight gain progress was slow, it was steady. Over the next few months I noticed that my skin started to look brighter, my clothes didn't bag as much on me, and I had more energy. I even started to exercise more regularly, which made me feel both stronger and hungrier—two sensations that had been missing for quite a while. For the first time in my life, I experienced gaining weight as a joy and not a catastrophe, because I knew that I was doing it on purpose and for the right reasons, as opposed to gaining weight as a result of being anxious and out of control with binging and purging.

I also took Annie's advice and started to reach out to her and my Baltimore program friends more actively instead of stewing in my sadness. I called and told them the truth about Renewal and its marginal chances for success. Instead of pushing away their sympathy, I allowed myself to take in their sorrow about the plight that Haywood and I were in, and shared my fears about how I didn't know how we would eventually get out of our financial hole.

Whenever I hung up the phone from these cathartic conversations I temporarily felt better, and even if our situation with Renewal remained unchanged, I temporarily behaved in a more upbeat and proactive way because of the healing power of talking honestly and being open. What made the conversations hard though, was that none of them had ever fallen so far, so fast, with their fortunes, and it was hard for them to grasp what we were dealing with, or to know what to say. So while I benefited from the calls, and enjoyed feeling connected to what was going on in others' lives, I still felt like I was experiencing something that they couldn't comprehend or empathize with.

Some unexpectedly nice things happened to me at this time, which gave me a small vacation from figuring out what we were going to do if Renewal went under. I was in my office one afternoon when the phone rang and a woman asked if she was talking to "the Caroline Miller who wrote that great book on bulimia."

Immediately puffed up, I promised her that I was, indeed, "that" Caroline Miller. "Can I help you?" I asked happily.

"I'm a producer for the show 'To Tell the Truth,'" she began, "and we read a story about you in a women's magazine that featured an excerpt from your book. We think you'd be the perfect guest for us, and we'd love to fly you out to Hollywood for a show where you would tell your story, and train two imposters to try to fool the celebrity judges about who the "real Caroline Miller" is."

I lit up. "Are you the same show where people pretend to stand up at the end, and they fake back and forth until the 'real' person stands up?"

I had clear memories of watching this show on our family's black and white television when I was a kid, and my favorite part had always been when the celebrity judges were proven right or wrong and the "real" person stood up. I immediately wanted to see how good I could be at pretending not to be me for once. It also made me smile to even think about having that kind of fun, which I hadn't had in quite some time.

"That's us, indeed!" The producer was delighted that she didn't have to explain the concept. Every episode started with three people in shadow, and the announcer's voice would boom, "Number One... what is your name, please?" The lights would explode on the person and they would say that their name was Joe Palooka, or whoever they were supposed to be, and this would be repeated two more times.

Then the three candidates would walk down the steps to a table where they would entertain probing questions about their life and accomplishments from a panel of celebrity judges. When time ran out, the judges would have to vote for who they thought the "real" person was, based on the answers they had gotten from the contestants, which was when the faking and dodging occurred.

Not only did "To Tell the Truth" turn out to be a lot of fun, it was also the first time I'd ever been away from my son. I did feel vaguely guilty as I departed, but it was also pretty nice not to have a diaper bag slung over my shoulder, or a bottle of formula in my purse. Being a full-time mom of an infant also meant that my senses were always on hyperalert, scanning the environment for possible danger, so dropping my vigilant stance for a few days was a relief. Wearing something other than jeans or a sweat suit stained with baby food and formula also reminded me that it was nice to dress up and be an interesting, attractive adult woman.

I felt like an animal sprung from a cage after I checked into my hotel near the television studios in Hollywood. Prowling the streets near my hotel, I soaked up a world of different smells, sounds and people than I'd experienced in my recent years of bulimia recovery, book tours, pregnancy, and business pressures. I felt giddy, intoxicated and free.

The next two days were spent helping two young women learn how to answer questions about bulimia and pretend to be me. The three of us ate together, laughed about the experience of trying to become someone else for a day, and I taught them about my life and my book. When the actual taping occurred, my imposters did such a great job that they got three of the four votes as being the "real" Caroline Miller, while I only got one, earning me a much-needed check for $750.

On the way home from my "To Tell the Truth" experience, I reflected on how much I had enjoyed being briefly away from my daily responsibilities, and how good it felt to be reminded about the power of my book, which had gotten lost in the shuffle of watching Renewal go under. I was also struck by how relieved I'd been to have a break from parenting for 48 hours, and how just being with other adults in a new setting, talking about a wide variety of topics, felt so healing. I needed more of this—laughter, distraction and money—but I didn't have that waiting for me at home, unfortunately.

\* \* \* \* \* \* \* \*

BACK IN MIDDLETOWN, I immediately felt isolated and lonely again. The town was still a foreign world to me, and I felt shy and uncertain about reaching out in my new environment to make friends I could actually meet on a regular basis without driving an hour or being on the telephone. I attended a few 12-step meetings in the community as a start, but they were sparse and poorly attended, which reminded me to be grateful that I had recovered in the vibrant city of Baltimore, where support group meetings were strong and plentiful.

Meeting other young moms wasn't as easy as I thought because Haywood was too young to be in a preschool or playgroup where that type of bonding often occurs naturally. We also didn't know how much longer we'd even be in the Middletown area, so my incentive to find outlets was minimal at best.

As a native Washingtonian, I had often noticed that foreigners who were temporarily stationed in the city's embassies would keep to themselves because they knew they'd be leaving within a few years, and it was too painful for them to say hello and goodbye to new friends over and over. I now understood their reticence to connect prior to the inescapable reality that they would soon be leaving again, so I stayed in my cocoon in the treatment center with my husband, son and telephone, uncertain of when we'd be able to escape ourselves.

My husband remained my primary in-person support system during the day, and somehow he always managed to make me smile, or we would do something goofy with our son to relieve the stress. Our daily mutual support sessions were waning, though, because he was increasingly leaving Middletown to interview for jobs in the Washington and Baltimore areas. Haywood and I had decided that we couldn't afford to live on our dreams any longer. So he began the painful process of calling all of our friends and acquaintances to tell them that he was throwing in the towel on our venture for good, and that he desperately needed a job to support his family.

It turned out that our dire situation contained at least one silver lining that helped Haywood in his job search. Prior to Renewal, he had been a corporate, white collar lawyer who did mind-numbing work like checking for missing commas in documents. Now his resumé reflected a person who had created a company, raised money, dealt with investors and banks, and knew a tremendous amount about the realities of running a for-profit organization and meeting payroll, however briefly. Many of the venture companies that he interviewed with were impressed that he wasn't a newly-minted MBA with nothing but classroom or book knowledge, and that he had actually taken a risk and gotten his hands dirty in the real world of running a business.

"You're just the kind of guy we need here," Haywood heard one euphoric day in late 1989, when he was offered a position with a publicly- traded venture fund in the Washington, D.C., suburbs. We were now so accustomed to hearing bad news that we waited to celebrate his good fortune until the offer was in writing and family healthcare insurance was guaranteed. Our merry band of three—me, my six-month old son and my husband—breathed our first sigh of relief in months as we gaily dined at the local Outback Steakhouse, which was an extravagant outing for us.

The news of Haywood's job couldn't have come at a better time. As delighted as I was for Haywood and our family's prospects, though, I acutely felt the loss of his supportive presence when he immediately began the long daily commute to and from Washington. Although we'd both been morose about our situation, we'd had each other to commiserate with during the long days of failed meetings and dashed hopes. Now I was abruptly left alone with a gurgling infant in an icy mansion for fourteen hours a day. I still had the support of my program friends on the telephone, but it simply wasn't enough to counteract the sad feelings that continued to engulf me whenever I had time to think about our situation.

Haywood's new job also decisively destroyed any lingering, irrational hopes I'd had that Renewal might get a last-minute savior. If he wasn't available any longer to negotiate with potential investors about our company, we had no conceivable hope of surviving. So as I watched his car pull away every morning at the crack of dawn, it finally and decisively hit me that my dream of creating a healing place for people with eating disorders was dead. I'd known for months that we were all but doomed, but now I had to accept complete defeat while still living in the shell of the center, which had begun to feel like a mausoleum.

Facing this was much harder than I had expected, particularly on one memorable gray day as I watched the Evergreen Renewal Center get auctioned off before my eyes. Hidden behind the curtains of our bedroom window so that people couldn't see me or witness my pain, I observed as an auctioneer representing the bank unsuccessfully attempted to raise enough money to cover their investment.

Despite my admonitions to myself not to get upset, I couldn't help feeling sad as I heard the auctioneer, representing the bank, throw out the minimum bid.

600,000 Dollars! Do I hear a bid for 600,000 dollars to get things rolling today?"

Although the figure represented the bank's financial liability, it was nowhere near the amount that we'd paid two years earlier for this property, not to mention the hundreds of thousands of dollars of improvements we'd put into it too. Real estate had gone into a freefall since we'd purchased and improved Two Sons Farm, though, so the bank was just hoping to recoup their investment. The timing couldn't have been worse for that to happen.

"600,000 Dollars! Do I hear 600,000 dollars?"

The auctioneer called out the figure repeatedly from his perch atop a box near the pond, but the gaggle of men and women who had come in an attempt to get our one-of-a-kind property for a bargain didn't make a move.

"It's just business," I reminded myself over and over as I saw people jostling each other and gazing longingly at the impressive building and surroundings.

"Going once, going twice, sold for $600,000!" The gavel came down with a loud clang.

The auction ended as quickly as it started. Without anyone offering the minimum bid and unwilling to stomach a massive loss, the bank bought the property back for itself. The crowd began to disperse.

I looked at the phone. I wanted to call Haywood to tell him that the auction had ended without success, but I didn't want to bother him. He needed to focus on his own work and his new future, and this development could wait for tonight. I thought about calling someone else, but I felt too raw and numb to reach out.

I stood up and walked into the bathroom to gather my thoughts. I stared at the mirror, somehow thinking that looking at my image would tell me what to do and how to regain my equilibrium. I didn't have any epiphany, but I did note that—unlike the scene several months earlier—I didn't look haunted and thin any longer. I did, however, still look incredibly sad, which was underscored by what I had just witnessed.

Not only did I look sad, but I looked cold, which never helped my mood. Looking into the mirror in this bathroom had been the impetus to challenge myself about my low weight months earlier, and I had now beaten it back. I had reached out to a role model who had helped me regain my footing with my food and body image, and the result was that I felt strong and steady in that area again.

But something was still missing. With no local friends, no job, and no distractions from my grim situation, I was alone most of the time, except for my baby, who hadn't proven to be a great conversationalist yet. My sleep was erratic and I had no real professional goals anymore, particularly in light of the final demise of our company today. Haywood was hitting his stride again in life, setting fresh resolutions based on his new line of work and beginning to visualize an exciting professional future, but I felt left behind.

What was I going to do? What kind of job could I get, and where? These questions were hard to answer.

I knew I needed to recapture some of my old zest and can-do spirit, but I was beginning to feel like that was going to be hard to pull off in this current conundrum. My contact with my program friends helped up to a point, but it seemed to just be a quick fix because I couldn't forestall the feelings of sadness and personal failure that always returned with a vengeance. Now the finality of the auction was going to unleash a new set of upsetting realities. Could I weather them by just calling Annie and others like her every day or so, hoping that they could invoke program slogans to help me slog through my troubles?

Although I had found that meetings and recovering people had had the power to help me transform myself and my life as I had overcome bulimia, I didn't feel like it was going to be enough to slay the current mental dragons I was up against. This felt bigger, deeper and blacker than anything I'd experienced before, and it was beginning to scare me.

I gazed back at myself in an unfocused, blank way. Minutes crept by as my mind filled with negative thoughts and pessimistic scenarios of future failure. Haywood would move ahead and be successful and I'd be the pathetic bulimic who had failed on a massive scale, and who had become well-known for something that most people found disgusting. People were probably laughing at me now, I thought darkly. The whole world was glad I had been so publicly humiliated because no one liked me, anyway. The familiar quicksand of depression was quickly enveloping me, clogging my brain and making clear thinking impossible.

I fiercely shook my head to return to reality, instead focusing on the features of my face, searching every freckle, angle and curve for answers. Through the other closed bathroom door I heard my son begin to move and make sounds. My heart melted. I loved him so much that it hurt at times. I wanted to make him proud, and sitting here in this cold bathroom, sadly ruminating about my lost dreams and spinning out dark fantasies, wouldn't help either of us.

I needed to be active. That had always been the answer to my problems before—stirring myself out of apathy and isolation by humbling myself, asking for help, setting goals and going after them, one day at a time.

I suddenly knew what I had to do to get started. And I couldn't act a moment too soon.

# CHAPTER EIGHT
## THE GOOD MOM

The therapist I'd seen when I first started my recovery five years earlier was retired, so I called one who had facilitated a women's empowerment group that I had attended just prior to getting pregnant. At that time, I had been upbeat about my book, my recovery and my plans for Renewal. Kathleen Martin had been one of the people in that gathering, and she had impressed me with her directness, humor, and ability to easily connect with others. I needed all of those qualities in a therapist, and I figured that if she wasn't the right person to see me now as a client, she would know who to recommend.

"Hi, this is Caroline Miller," I said to her answering machine. "I met you in a women's group two years ago. Since then, I've had a baby and moved to Middletown. Life isn't going very well for me right now. I feel sad most of the time and I'm embarrassed to admit it, given the fact I've written a book about recovery from bulimia and I've presented myself to the world as a healthy and high-functioning woman. If you think the type of therapy you do would be helpful, would you call me back?"

A couple of hours later, Kathleen returned my call and I shared a few more details about my life and why I was reaching out to her. We agreed to meet to determine if more therapy was what I actually needed again, and whether or not her philosophy and approach would work for me. I wasn't surprised that I felt more hopeful simply because I'd made this call, because that had been my pattern since hitting my last bottom in 1984. Whenever I was desperate and reached out, my mood immediately spiked because the sheer action of admitting that I needed support and guidance gave me a powerful high, as well as the hope that change was already underway.

Our son had never been left alone with anyone except a family member, so finding someone to watch him in Middletown for a few hours required a few calls to inquire about local childcare resources. Luckily, the daughter-in-law of our immediate neighbor ran a small family daycare service on her farm a mile or so away, and she was delighted to take Haywood for an afternoon later that week while I drove an hour each way to meet with Kathleen.

Sherri was younger than me, but had three children who were already adolescents because she had started her family at a very young age. A farmer's life is one of relentless, hard work, but Sherri was contagiously upbeat and bubbly, starting with her smile. She disarmed my young son instantly by greeting him at the car door and telling him that he was going to go with her to feed the goats in the barn. Without a whimper, Haywood smiled happily as she hefted him into her arms. He didn't even look back as I slowly drove away.

Just as I'd felt on the day I left for "To Tell the Truth" in California, I was caught between feeling guilty and relieved as I got onto the interstate highway and realized that I didn't have to care for an infant for the next few hours, and that I could just focus on myself. My feelings of guilt about not being totally preoccupied with my son at all times clearly had deep roots I needed to untangle. When I was young, I remembered learning that my mother had given up a reporting career at the *Washington Post* to be a stay-at-home mom to my brother, sister and myself. Instead of pursuing a rewarding career with her writing talents, she chose to cook, clean, drive carpools and spend every waking moment taking care of our needs, not taking a job again until I was in college to help pay for the various school tuitions.

I couldn't remember many occasions where my grandmother wasn't our babysitter, either, so I had internalized the message that "good" moms stayed home, took care of their families, and did little for themselves and that the babysitting pool extended only to immediate family. "Bad" moms worked and didn't truly love their children because random, uncaring sitters raised them. As I drove to Kathleen's appointment, I mused that I couldn't even remember seeing my mom get a manicure, have a bunch of girlfriends over for a party, or take a vacation by herself.

Had this life made her happy? I didn't know, but I didn't think it had. In fact, I now believed that being a full-time mom all of those years had brought out the worst in her, possibly without her even realizing how much she was taking her unhappiness out on her children. Had she had serious dreams at one point about what she longed to accomplish in her own life? If so, I had no idea what they were. Maybe she hadn't had goals, or even felt permitted to have them.

Furthermore, I'd rarely seen my mother have fun or even laugh spontaneously. Her workmanlike approach to life had been inculcated into us as children as far as how to live our own lives. I had unquestioningly followed orders, working hard in private schools, swim practices, playing the piano, and doing everything asked of me so that I could achieve a standard of excellence. I couldn't honestly say that I'd ever had fun either. Everything had been competitive or sheer hard work.

It was beginning to make sense to me why enjoying being away from my child for a few stolen hours didn't come naturally to me. I wondered if I would ever have the capacity to be like my husband and spend an entire day at work, never wondering if he was a "bad" parent.

And what was Haywood's opinion of leaving his son with a babysitter so that I could work? I realized that we'd never really talked about it in earnest, although we both had expressed a preference for one parent to be with him as much as possible. Would my husband be angry if I made the choice to work outside the home? And if he were, would I have the courage to pursue a job that would give me a break from the tedium of motherhood while also contributing to the family's busted finances? Like me, Haywood had been raised in a home where women simply weren't expected to work, and child-rearing was considered the epitome of success. But was that going to completely fulfill *me*?

I wondered about this and other issues as I made the fifty-mile journey to Kathleen's office and sorted through what I wanted to cover in our time together. Instead of overwhelming her with the enormity of how I felt about our financial challenges, I wanted to focus on some of the things that were dogging me from day to day—loneliness, feelings of inadequacy and failure around Renewal's demise.

Finally, I felt emotionally numb. Nothing seemed to make me happy for any significant length of time, and I didn't feel like I had anything to look forward to. Intellectually, I knew that this was ridiculous, given that I had a healthy child who would undoubtedly grow up and fill my life with delight, and a husband who loved me. My miserable perceptions of my current and future life, however, were proof of just how depressed and pessimistic I had become.

* * * * * * * *

KATHLEEN'S WAITING ROOM featured a blend of burbling water, neutral paintings, several clocks, and soft chairs. Personal touches were absent. I was always amused by this type of professional bland decorating that was designed to avoid provoking any strong emotions, one way or the other. In a perverse way, it had always led me to secretly want to say or do something outrageous, just to break the spell of forced sanity.

I had only been seated for a moment when Kathleen opened her door and greeted me with warmth and a gentle embrace.

"I'm glad you came," she said as she led me into her softly-lit and tranquil office.

"So would you like to elaborate a bit more about what's happening in your life and why you felt the need to call me?" Kathleen began, settling into an oversized chair opposite my own voluminous chair.

"I'm just feeling awful." That was all it took for the tears to start. Somehow, just beginning this dialogue and not needing to be a strong, brave, recovered person or vigilant mom, opened the floodgates.

We spent the next hour getting reacquainted as I brought her up to speed on my life, my concerns, and some of my recent worries about being too thin. The time flew by too quickly, but I felt the familiar balm of healing from speaking openly.

At the end of the hour, Kathleen asked, "Have you ever been diagnosed with depression?"

I shook my head. "No. In fact, I've always been told that I come across as pretty together, particularly because I had to fight so hard to just get better from the bulimia. And I don't think I've ever been this sad before, either. It's like a quicksand that sucks me in if I'm alone for too long, or I have too much bad news all at once. Is that full-blown depression, or just the result of living a depressing life right now?"

"I don't know," Kathleen replied. "It could be both. But just from what you've shared with me, you might have had an underlying depression that predated the eating disorder and has genetic roots, and that has been reactivated because of the bankruptcy, hormonal fluctuations, and major disruptions to your life. And if I were to look at the list of top ten stressors, I'd guess that you had at least seven of them happen to you in just one year. That would be enough to knock anyone out of the box, regardless of any predisposition to depression."

"So how would I know which one it is? Or if it's both?"

"We'd have to watch that together, if you decided to work with me. And if some of our work didn't significantly lessen your feelings of shame or sadness, I'd want you to be evaluated by a psychiatrist who specializes in medication to see if an anti-depressant might help you regain your emotional footing more quickly."

I didn't reply immediately. Although Haywood was on medication for his epilepsy, which had been diagnosed during the first year of our marriage after a number of *petit mal* and *grand mal* seizures, I had some strong feelings about the idea of going on a drug to change or enhance my well being. Couldn't I just work a little harder to improve my mood? Somehow, it felt like yet another prospect of seeing myself as a failure if I had to take a pill to be a happier person.

"Can I just think about it?" I finally responded. "I'm not sure I'm ready for that step."

"Absolutely," Kathleen said. "But my professional opinion is that you are probably clinically depressed, and seeing me at least once a week would be the least you could do to take control of your life and emotions. Twice a week would be preferable, but I know funds are tight, so I'd like to offer to see you at a deeply discounted fee and have you reimburse me when you are back on your feet."

Although I knew I needed this type of professional guidance, I told Kathleen that it was hard for me to feel like I deserved her generous offer. Outside of the volunteer help and support that I'd gotten in my support groups, accepting anything else from others was very hard for me because I had always felt like I had to earn the right to receive kindness from anyone. On Thanksgiving, I told Kathleen, I'd been taken aback to find that the construction company that had renovated the property but now would never get paid, had dropped off a turkey dinner for us. It had surprised and touched me because although the company owners didn't know us well, they still knew that we were in dire straits and they wanted to reach out to make our holiday a little brighter.

"Why did that surprise you?" Kathleen looked at me quizzically. As she posed the question, I instantly knew that my answer would probably contain some seeds of insight into why I was in this tough place.

Without missing a beat I said, "Because I don't think I'm worthy of it."

As I answered the question I flashed back to my first night in the eating disorder self-help group in February 1984 where I sat mute, angry and unapproachable at the back of a room, knowing I needed help but upset that I'd had to go to a church basement at night to get it from strangers. I had eventually let the group's members into my life and my heart, and I had given generously to them, too. But despite these experiences, I still found my tough exterior and "I can take care of myself" attitude coming out at times, along with my pride.

Kathleen smiled sympathetically. "We need to work on that. If you don't think you're truly worthy of kindness and generosity from others, you will find ways to punish yourself and shut others out. This will feed into your loneliness and keep you separated from people who want to nurture and support you in your time of need."

We agreed to meet twice a week for the foreseeable future on a sliding scale. Kathleen asked me to keep an open mind about entering group therapy with her at some point, because it was apparent that there was a disconnect between how others perceived me and how I perceived myself. She noted that our individual work could only go so far in addressing that issue, but that the dynamics of being in a group would flush these and other topics out into the open to be examined.

I smiled and sang along with the radio as I made the long drive back to Middletown. Once again, nothing had changed, but *everything* had changed because I had reached out for help with the earnest desire to examine myself and address whatever was standing between me and happiness. I'd done it six years earlier when I thought my life had hung in the balance because of bulimia, and I'd miraculously gotten better. And although I didn't know where this particular step back into therapy was going to ultimately take me, my inner neon sign had just flashed "Right Way!" I trusted it enough at this point to just follow.

# CHAPTER NINE
## "THE BAD SEED"

For the next few months, Kathleen and I focused on a few specific areas so I could get some emotional and financial traction in my life. Of special interest was identifying the self-defeating thoughts and behaviors that prevented me from being more resilient in the face of setbacks. Our first job had been addressing the "good mom" emotional quagmire by finding some type of gainful employment that didn't require being away from my child more than a few hours a day. Haywood had been happy with his hours at Sherri's farm, plus he'd gotten to socialize with other children, so that gave me a safe base from which to flex what remained of my professional muscles. Fortunately, my agent was able to get me another book contract based on the success of my first one; thus was born *Feeding the Soul*, a daily meditation book for people suffering from eating disorders. I settled into a familiar rhythm of morning writing while Haywood was at daycare and then picked him up after his nap so I could spend the rest of the day with him. It felt right.

"You seem happier," Kathleen remarked one day as I settled into my familiar spot in her office.

"I am, but it still comes and goes more often than I'd like," I answered. "Although I'm writing a new book and continuing to run my non-profit, we're so far behind the eight ball financially that I can't really see the light at the end of the tunnel yet. Haywood has worked out repayment deals now with our creditors, and I'm glad he has a job, but I'm still ashamed of where we are financially, and how much money we lost for other people who believed in us. I almost feel like when the center died, it killed a piece of me, too."

"So the center was *you*? And if it wasn't successful, you aren't worth anything? Do you always have to win at everything you do?"

I squirmed. It sounded kind of pathetic. I hadn't thought about it this way, but when Kathleen said it, it made sense. Our sessions were like twice-weekly archaeological excavations; we always started with a statement I made about something on my mind, and then we followed it until we hit the payoff of a fresh and useful insight. I digested each new awareness, getting fresh footholds to build different behaviors and better ways of thinking. Like gaining weight, the progress was incredibly slow, but steady.

"Yes, I guess I lost sight of who I was in the process of being so public with the book and then with the treatment center. Everything became completely personal and on a national stage, and I can't seem to always separate what happened to Renewal from what has happened to me."

"So who are you if you're not achieving something or proving your worth financially to others?"

"I don't know. I guess I don't see myself as valuable unless I'm successful at whatever I'm working on. It's pretty black and white for me." I hadn't really known how extreme these views were until the words actually came out of my mouth. Therapy had a way of making me have and express the irrational beliefs that were lurking somewhere inside me, but that had no way to escape until I was asked a question in a certain way, and in a supportive setting.

"Tell me about yourself. What do you like about yourself?"

I was silent. I didn't know what to say. I didn't know that I actually liked a whole lot about myself, but I was eloquent about everything I thought was broken. THAT was an easy question to answer, so I started there.

"Maybe I can answer by telling you what I don't like, and we can figure out what's missing," I began. "I'm critical, I hold grudges, I'm disorganized, moody, broke…"

"Stop!" Kathleen commanded. "Tell me one thing about yourself that is good, that has nothing to do with a weakness. You have to be able to think of something, or I'm going to wonder what we've been doing for months together."

Again, I was quiet, but what came to mind was a line from a diary I had started in seventh grade in which I described what I looked like. I had written, "My eyes are my best feature." I had no idea why I had written that, but it had been prior to the onset of my eating disorder, which was when my self-loathing had started. At one time, though, I had had the self-confidence to say that I actually liked something about myself. I wasn't sure a positive thought had crossed my brain for many years after that moment.

"My eyes," I finally admitted, stealing an idea from my old diary, but embellishing it with what I hoped sounded like a useful insight. "I like my eyes, but I think that's because I'm good at reading people. I am rarely wrong about someone's character, good or bad, which is why I love watching people. I take in everything about them and use my intuition to help me gauge what they are really like and whether or not I can trust them."

"That's a start," Kathleen admitted, "but can you see how hard it is for you to even come up with that one thing, and how you continue to put a low value on yourself unless you're a Harvard graduate, book author, or successful businesswoman? Can you see that your concept of your self-worth, much of it resulting from how you were raised, has been so tied to success and winning that it took one massive "failure," as you describe it, to make you devalue everything good about yourself? How about the fact that you're resilient and gutsy? That you had the nerve to tell the world a story about yourself that others might have found shameful? Or that you are a hard worker, and you give 100% to everything you do? Or that you are smart and curious about people and life? What about the incredible love you have for your son? I have only known you for a short period, but those are obvious qualities that jump out at me."

It was nice to hear her compliment me, but the negatives still loomed larger to me, and I told her so.

"How do I learn to consistently—not occasionally—value myself as something other than what I appear to be externally? I intellectually understand what you're saying and why you're saying it, but I don't think I know how to do it and stay in that place."

"Aha! You need to begin to observe and honor who you are inside, and treasure the moments when you are kind, or compassionate, or committed, and not simply put a price tag on the externals. Savor those moments and replay them, don't let them just pass you by without honoring them. You will find yourself vulnerable to the judgments of others if you only focus on superficial things that can come and go, like possessions, money, houses and looks."

Kathleen leaned forward to emphasize her point. "Caroline, it's not about your *doing* that makes you worthwhile. It's about your *being* that makes you who you are."

We explored more about where I had learned that externals mattered more than internals, which dated back to my childhood and the pressures to be successful in a competitive town like Washington, D.C. Getting into the right preschool, and then the right elementary school, and then the right high school was the ticket to acceptance in the community I lived in, and the bumper stickers on your car told the story about whether or not your child measured up.

It was also clear to me now that I'd only felt valuable to my parents if I'd been "the best" in something, or if I'd had some type of success they could talk about. Otherwise, my mother repeatedly told me that I was a "bad" person, and that others could see it just by looking at me. On a number of occasions, she would pull up next to a car in traffic, and point to the driver of the other car and say, "See that person? They know what you're really like because of how ugly you are being with me." Once, when I was on my way to a birthday party in fifth grade, she held up one of my favorite dresses—a black frilly dress with fat, pink roses all over it—and said, "Here, put on your costume to cover up who you really are." The message was always clear: Caroline was bad and everyone else was better. The only brief reprieves came if I actually was temporarily "the best" at something, which allowed them to bask in my reflected glory. The problem is that being "the best" never lasts, regardless of who you are.

Divulging these stories to Kathleen over many months, and processing many of them for the first time since they'd occurred almost twenty years earlier, was the painful price I had to pay to plumb the roots of my low self-esteem, and learn how to face life more resiliently. Looking back on the therapy I'd done just as I began to deal with my eating disorder, I saw that it had just been the tip of the iceberg. Now I was going much deeper.

One afternoon, as Kathleen and I discussed the fact that I stayed away from many people out of a fear that I would bring nothing of value to the relationship, I told her something I had never told anyone else and that haunted me even as an adult.

"When I was around eleven or twelve, a well-known author published a book of short stories, and because we had other books by this author, my parents bought the book and began to pass it around the family." I licked my lips as I felt my familiar feelings of shame rise.

"The first story in the book was called 'The Bad Seed.' "One night I heard my parents and my sister laughing about the name of that story in the kitchen, which was directly below my bedroom." The tears welled up as I tumbled backwards in time and became that sad, picked-on girl again.

"That's Caroline—she's our bad seed," my dad said gaily, loud enough for me to hear fresh peals of laughter in my bedroom.

Up in my room, hearing the family discuss me in this way, I'd felt sick and humiliated. It had further cemented the outsider status I had felt in my own family since I was very young, and that lots of other people had commented on as I'd grown up. "You don't really fit in," my college roommates and others had often said. "You're so… different."

Being described as "the bad seed" hurt me more deeply than anything my parents had ever said or done up until that point. Years later, that phrase had been used as the description of the Devil's spawn, Damien, in the horror flick, "The Omen." When that movie became the rage in 1976, a year or so after my eating disorder had taken hold of my body and soul, all I could think was that God didn't love me because I was "the bad seed," and that my eating disorder was my punishment for having the Devil inside me.

And if God didn't love me and my parents didn't love me, would anyone ever really love me? And could I ever fully love myself if I'd never been raised with authentic and unconditional love in my home? My first therapist had once remarked that given the lack of expressed love in the house, including the omission of all touch and kissing, it was remarkable that I'd been able to forge a bond with anyone. My grandmother's fierce and unconditional love for me had clearly been the lifeline that saved me and gave me hope.

Kathleen saw how this revelation was starting to carry me away with emotion. She firmly brought me back into the room to deal with it instead of just reacting to it. "How did that feel to hear your family talk about you as the bad seed?" She probed with firm, but kind, words.

"Horrible. But I felt like somehow I deserved it," I answered softly, lowering my head and letting the hot tears burn my face.

I felt dirty, young and homeless sitting in front of this middle-aged woman, even though that episode had occurred fifteen years earlier and I was now safe. The tears I cried for several minutes were angry and gut-wrenching. Instead of experiencing and processing my grief when these types of events had happened as a child, I had learned to turn on myself, instead. I knew that no one would ever believe me if I shared these stories, and I'd never had anyone to turn to, anyway, outside of my grandmother. The bulimia had become my only escape because the numbness brought on by the purges disconnected me briefly from the world, much the same way an alcoholic uses booze to anesthetize feelings.

I stopped crying long enough to finish my story. "I never touched that short story book. I can still see the red cover and where it sat in our family's den. And just hearing the words, 'the bad seed,' is still enough to cause my throat to choke up and my confidence to go away now," I admitted. "I was treated as the bad seed all the time, no matter what I said, did or achieved. I tried so hard to be successful so that they would stop, but it never stopped. And I never understood what I did to cause it all to start, either."

I looked at Kathleen. "I don't think I really believed that I could be loved or even wanted as a friend when I was younger." I didn't want to tell her that I had asked Haywood to marry me on our third date in college because I'd been afraid that no one else would ever ask me out again. Thankfully, he'd had his own reasons to want to rush into this adult commitment, so two years later we'd tied the knot at the ridiculously young ages of 21 and 23. But had that been love? Would the emotions that led us to be together have the depth to withstand all of the tests coming at us now? I guess I was going to find out.

Because there were no easy answers to these questions, Kathleen just let them hang in the air, suspended like icicles. The enormity of what I had just relived, shared and was clearly still struggling with, was apparent. Although I was close to thirty years old and an adult by most measures, I had reverted once again to feeling like a wounded child who had nowhere to turn for love or understanding.

"That's more than enough for one day." Kathleen rose and gave me a hug. "All I can say is that I'm very sorry you had to go through this. Your task now is to learn to love yourself in spite of what was done to you. When you heal, you will eventually learn how to really trust and love other people, too. That, my dear, is when you will know happiness that doesn't come and go."

I hugged Kathleen a little bit harder and longer before I let go and went out to my car. I was exhausted by the revelations. Parenting was not a gig to be entrusted to just anyone, I thought as I gathered my thoughts before starting the long drive back to Middletown. Had my parents thought they were doing a great job with me? Why hadn't they gone to a shrink to talk about whether or not my "badness" was real or imagined? And why was I, the one with no resources, spending money to undo the damage now?

Clearly, if I was going to experience any type of lasting inner joy, it wasn't going to come from having a house, money, healthy children or a fit body that didn't suffer from bulimia. No, I could really see that while all of those things would contribute to my peace of mind, my primary job at this point in my life was to learn how to just be Caroline—whoever that was—and to love her no matter what.

## CHAPTER TEN
## THE WILLY WONKA GOLDEN TICKET

Although the holiday was months away, my husband had snagged an item that he felt would make the day special.

"Look!" he exclaimed as he greeted us one night after work. He held up a tiny green sweatshirt with dragon scales that ran from the hood down the back. "This is Haywood's first Halloween costume!"

I had laughed, thinking about our two-and-a-half-year-old ball of fire in a green dragon suit, going door-to-door asking for candy. This immediately started me thinking about some of my favorite childhood memories of exuberant Halloween nights with my best friend, Anne Ginsburgh, whose internal motor had easily been as powerful as mine. Together, we had trick-or-treated every year from kindergarten through eighth grade, at which time we reluctantly decided we were too old for such immature things.

Anne and I had discovered each other on the playground when we were both five, and we bonded instantly and caroused famously for years. Our innate zest, athletic interests and constant chattering had bedeviled a number of teachers who didn't know how to contain our energy levels—magnified when we were together—so we had been deliberately separated and put into different classrooms from the age of six onwards. News of our personalities had preceded our arrival at Washington's National Cathedral School for Girls, our home for the next nine years. The teachers separated us there too, which was probably wise, even though it never lessened our desire to make merry and be loud.

One of the painful legacies of my bulimia was that I had begun to pull away from people like Anne when my eating disorder absorbed my life in ninth grade. Instead of nurturing friendships and relying on my "tribe" during the turbulent teen years, I often stayed at home alone, miserable about my body and self-destructive behavior, but too scared to tell anyone or ask for help. As a result, Anne and others drifted away, unable to comprehend who I had become.

Later, when I rigorously went through the list of people I wanted to apologize to as part of my recovery, Anne had been one of the first amends letter I'd written. I'd explained what had happened to me, and how the bulimia had sucked me so far under for so many years that I'd been unable to reach out for help to her or anyone else. I had dearly missed our closeness, I wrote, but like many other things, the bulimia had left no room in my life for anything good.

Anne had been more than happy to meet me halfway as an adult woman and try to understand what had happened to me, but we were never able to recreate our close bond. Too many years had gone by.

Kathleen and I had begun to explore the impact of being isolated during the years when people traditionally learn how to navigate the social scene and learn friendship skills, along with constantly being told by my parents that I wasn't a good, worthy person.

"It's like the Leaning Tower of Pisa," she noted one day when we were talking about learning how to bond with others and be in healthy relationships. "Depending on where you are in the life cycle, you'll be looking at this issue from a different floor as you go around and around the Tower. You'll be able to address certain facets while looking out one window, and a few years later, you may see a new angle from a higher floor that has to be addressed. It's a lifelong journey with things like this, but one that you'll always be making progress on if you continue to strive for growth and change."

Prior to the onset of the eating disorder and teenage friendship challenges, though, Anne and I had had a Halloween childhood ritual of racing through local neighborhoods with pillowcases that were, by evening's end, so full that we couldn't stuff another gumball in them. Then we'd collapse at her house or mine and paw through the piles of candy, trading what we didn't want, adding up how many Sugar Daddies or Milky Ways we had, and chewing on our sugary bounty until our teeth stuck together.

The idea of my son heading down this same annual road of fun memories, beginning with his dragon costume, delighted me. The only problem was that our new neighborhood only had four or five houses within walking distance and our street dead-ended at one of the most familiar sites around: a cornfield.

Despite this obvious Halloween limitation, though, I was happy to finally be in our own place again, free of the reminders of the treatment center that never was and would never be. As much as I'd wanted to have some resolution to how long we'd be living in the mansion, though, and living month to month at the mercy of our creditors, the denouement of our occupation there had occurred without warning, and we'd been given less than two weeks' notice to dismantle the remnants of the center, pack up our possessions, and find a place to live—which turned out to be just blocks from the center itself.

Although the house we'd moved into was quite small, it felt like heaven. We could barely afford it, but it worked for us. We had nice neighbors, many of them decades older and retired from long careers as postal workers or machinists. They smiled and waved when we met, we watched each other's pets when needed, and when there was a downed power line or someone required assistance, we connected in the middle of the street and pooled our resources.

Haywood still drove a long way to work every day, but I used the third bedroom for my writing while our son continued to grow into a happy and rambunctious little boy. We were in tremendous debt, and probably would be for another decade or more, but our household move put some emotional distance between us and Renewal's debacle, so we were healing in a number of ways.

Although Kathleen had proven to be a terrific therapist for me, alternately pushing and comforting me as I grappled with a variety of issues, the weekly sessions often left me reeling. Dredging up painful memories, connecting them with my current behaviors, and sharing them with someone else exhausted me.

If the topic was a deeply buried secret, I frequently felt like I'd opened Pandora's Box and let out all of the buzzing demons who then wouldn't leave me alone for days. Shaking off what was triggered in therapy became harder as we dug deeper and deeper, so Kathleen suggested that I revisit the issue of medication to see if something could help me bounce back a bit more quickly every time I picked off another emotional scab.

I trusted her judgment, especially after working together for over a year, so I agreed to visit the office of a psychiatrist who specialized in medication. I went to the appointment willingly but found that my lingering suspicions around medication were still very much alive. As hard as therapy was, I still enjoyed the rigorous process of turning myself inside out, realizing that I needed to do something different, and then struggling through the implementation of new thoughts and behaviors. It may have been somewhat Calvinistic, but I admired people who had the fortitude to survive and thrive in tough therapy. Taking a pill wasn't as admirable to me; anyone could do it, and short-cuts didn't impress me.

"Would you like to take your coat off?"

I sat across from Dr. Brown, arms crossed, coat on. He had noticed that I hadn't made myself comfortable, almost as if I didn't intend to stay.

"No, thanks."

I felt like I was at my first support group meeting for compulsive eaters. At that meeting seven years earlier I'd sat in the back row on a cold folding chair, arms folded defensively across my chest, a floppy bow-tie shirt and pearls serving as my armor to keep others away. Although I'd hit my last bottom that week by wretchedly binging and purging myself into a stupor, and knew I needed to be in that room to confess my powerlessness over food and what it did to me, I'd still been afraid to admit I needed help to anyone else. My loner "I can do it myself" attitude often collided with the little voice that told me to reach out. I usually ended up asking for help, but my independent side still came along as a silent partner.

"Are you depressed?"

Dr. Brown didn't mince words. He'd also been briefed by Kathleen beforehand, with my approval, so that we could make progress fast.

"I'm better than I was a year ago, but at times, I definitely struggle." I explained a bit about my eating disorder history, my challenge in getting pregnant, the four household moves I'd been through in two years, as well as the bankruptcy of Renewal.

Dr. Brown whistled. "Pretty impressive. That's a lot for anyone. Let me tell you a bit about how medication works, and why anti-depressants might be a good thing for you to try, given what Kathleen told me and what you have said today."

I began to relax a bit as Dr. Brown gave me a tutorial on the brain, reuptake inhibitors, serotonin, dopamine, and stress. I had always liked school, and this was a useful lesson, so I became absorbed in what he was saying.

"Given what I know about you, it's quite possible that your brain isn't manufacturing enough 'feel-good' chemicals at this point for you to hang onto what happiness you do have. This whole process may need to be jump-started so that your brain can learn how to make these chemicals for itself again."

That sounded accurate. I often felt that joy, or contented moments, didn't stay put with me. While my husband could usually put himself into a good mood, look for the bright side of a down situation, and stay there, it always felt like a hard slog for me.

"So what I'm suggesting is that you consider a medication trial to see if something might help to jumpstart the creation of the right chemicals in your brain, and then let them linger long enough in the right places to help you become happier."

Dr. Brown's idea sounded reasonable. "For how long?" I asked. "Is this the kind of thing people go on and never get off?"

He leaned back in his desk chair and put his fingers together in a steeple. "It really depends on you. Do you know if anyone in your family has ever been on depression medication, or had the diagnosis of depression?"

"Nope. I'm sure there is depression, but it's never been diagnosed that I know of. I also barely have any family at all to study. My parents were only children, and my grandmother was the only relative I ever knew. So without cousins, aunts, uncles or grandparents, I don't even think there is anyone to consult."

My grandmother, I wanted to tell him, wouldn't even allow the talk of depression in her presence because of her upbringing as a Christian Scientist. As much as I loved Donny, my mother's mother, her religion had always perplexed me because of the emphasis on denying bad things, which she called "errors." Trying to have a conversation about sickness, traumatic events or sad feelings was a word game with her.

"I don't feel good," I'd say to Donny when I was younger, and I had a stomach ache or wanted to use it as an excuse not to do something she wanted me to do.

"You are fine. There is no such thing as sickness," she would reply emphatically.

I often used the "I don't feel good" excuse when she took me out on our occasional trips to the Howard Johnson cafeteria, where she indulged me with roast beef and two desserts, as long as I would agree to eat some liver with bacon, which she always plopped onto my tray. "It's good for your blood," she'd explain, as she marched me through the line.

I tried my excuse again one night when I was about eight and told Donny that I felt sick. "I really don't think I can eat this," I said uneasily, as I eyed the mahogany-colored, leathery portion of liver swimming in thick gravy.

"There is no illness," she said again. "God is good. God wouldn't want you to feel bad. Try the liver. It will make you feel better."

I adored my grandmother, who was still alive, but we never made progress on my understanding of her viewpoint, or her agreeing that chicken pox might actually be a real sickness, so we'd just avoided this type of conversation and stayed on neutral territory in most of our conversations. She was getting older now, and was in her late eighties with a failing memory. The idea of asking her for data about her family around depression would obviously be laughable, because not only did depression not exist, Christian Scientists didn't take any medicine. So if I took medication for depression, that would be a double-negative error in Donny's book.

"Well if you don't have any information about depression in your family, or know of anyone else who has benefitted from being on an anti-depressant, we might want to start with Prozac, which acts on the sero-tonin pathways of the body and appears to impact the 'feel-good' pathways quickly and directly."

Dr. Brown gave me a bit more information about Prozac, which I'd certainly heard a lot about. This new medication had come out in the previous year, heralded by a huge smiley face on the cover of a news magazine.

I wanted to be a smiley face. I wanted to be the little girl I'd once been, tearing through neighborhoods with my best friend again, happy to just be silly and have fun for a night. I couldn't remember the last time I'd felt that way in any kind of lasting way. Probably before the eating disorder had started, and that was half a lifetime ago.

I pointed to the prescription pad in front of Dr. Brown. "I'll try Prozac." When I made a decision to move ahead with something, I was resolute. The neon sign inside my gut was flashing, "Right Way!" so I was impatient to get out of his office and get started with this trial.

"Prozac has a half-life of six weeks, so you won't get the full effect for at least a month," Dr. Brown cautioned, writing the prescription and handing it to me. "But I'd like you to be in touch with me over the next few weeks to let me know how you're doing."

I agreed and took the prescription. I was happy, once again, because I'd taken a risk and stepped outside my comfort zone to ask for help. Although I didn't know if this little piece of paper was going to be my ticket to feeling better on a consistent basis, I still felt like I had one of the five Golden Tickets from the Willy Wonka Chocolate bars, and I wanted to see what it was going to get me.

✳ ✳ ✳ ✳ ✳ ✳ ✳ ✳

"WHOOPS, SORRY..." my head snapped back up as I sat in Kathleen's comfortable fat chair, talking to her about Prozac. I'd been on it for less than two weeks, but I was not feeling happier yet. What I did feel, though, was much sleepier. Way sleepier. For a woman who'd always been known as somewhat frenetic, it was odd to find myself slipping away from my computer in the middle of the day to take a nap. Now, sitting in Kathleen's office in the middle of the day, I was surprising both of us by nodding off.

"Is this normal?" I asked.

"I don't think so," Kathleen frowned. "At least, I've never known that to be the case. You should let Dr. Brown know that you're usually more energetic than you're feeling on the medication. See what he says." I nodded. I was finding it harder and harder to stay awake, or feel motivated to follow through on anything I needed to do. Since starting Prozac I'd had a strange feeling of passivity but also wanted to collect a few more experiences before calling Dr. Brown with my feedback.

That decision was taken away from me within 24 hours, as I had no choice but to let him know what happened to me later that night.

"Oww..." I moaned from my side of the bed, suddenly feeling sharp pains in my abdomen. "Oww!" It felt like I was in labor, but that wasn't possible. I had one baby and it had to stay that way until we had some money in the bank. No getting pregnant for us now. I looked at the clock. It was just after 2 a.m.

I tried to turn over but I couldn't move without making the abdominal pains worse. "Haywood! Help!"

He instantly woke up and turned on the light.

"What? Is something wrong with Haywood?" He started to throw the covers off and move towards the door, only then realizing that I was the one in distress. It was funny how a parent's first thoughts, even in a deep sleep, are always about whether or not a child is okay.

He leaned over me, squinting. "What's wrong?"

"I don't know." I felt my stomach gently. Even that small movement hurt. "I think I need to go to the hospital. I don't know where my appendix is, but maybe I've burst it or something."

Hours later, I emerged from the local hospital Emergency Room with the diagnosis that I'd had a rare, but real, side-effect to the Prozac. I wasn't going to be a smiley face on this drug.

Dr. Brown and I faced off in his office later that week.

"Now what? Seems like I've failed at the most successful antidepressant of our time," I commented with a wry smile. "I thought I'd be a smiley face by now."

Dr. Brown wasn't amused. "Tell me as many details about your eating disorder recovery as you can," he said, pulling a legal pad in front of him. "When did your eating disorder start, how long did you suffer, and exactly how long have you been in recovery? And how do you know you're in recovery, anyway? What does that term mean to you? That you're better most of the time, but you have setbacks occasionally?"

It was actually refreshing to talk to someone who hadn't seen my story on television or read about it in the local papers. It was also an opportunity to put my recovery into words as I saw it today, and to let him know that it hadn't included any food setbacks for over five years.

After sharing the severity, duration and dates of my bulimia onset and the beginning of recovery, I told the doctor that I'd pieced together my recovery through a self-help group over several years, sticking with recovering people and using them as role models. I noted that I'd started with a small group of safe foods and had expanded that list as I'd trusted my body more, with pregnancy forcing me to further widen my palate. I added that I had stopped drinking alcohol years earlier, too, as a way of keeping myself from altering my mood in destructive ways and weakening my willpower.

"I don't worry about binging and purging, or even about overeating anymore," I said. "I consider myself completely recovered now. The Sword of Damocles isn't hanging over my head any longer."

Dr. Brown tapped his pen on his pad and looked me up and down. "You're slender," he finally said. "How can I trust that you're actually in the recovery you say you're in?"

I was momentarily shocked. He didn't believe me just because I wasn't heavy? What was eating disorder recovery supposed to look like anyway? I asked him that question.

"I don't know exactly," he replied, flustered. "But how would I know you were in recovery, other than what you're telling me? After all, you don't have any proof, other than what you say—right?"

I was getting angry. I had faced down this "you don't look like you're in recovery" challenge from another quarter within the last year, but certainly one of the most unexpected ones. After I'd addressed my issues around thinness with Annie, and before we'd been forced to leave the treatment center, I had been invited to meet with the owners of a Christian eating disorder treatment center. Despite its beautiful setting and trained personnel, the center was new and having trouble attracting enough clients to get on solid economic footing.

The center's founders had asked if I would be comfortable referring all interested Renewal applicants to them in exchange for a finder's fee. This had felt like manna in the wilderness, given our finances, and it would have also afforded me a way to help people find the residential treatment I couldn't offer them now. So I'd eagerly agreed to spend a day at their facility, to see if their philosophy matched the one espoused in my book and that I'd touted for Renewal, which they promised it did.

After a few hours of sitting in on meetings and therapy sessions, though, it was obvious that the center didn't adhere to a 12-step philosophy or even use it, and instead attacked eating disorders through a purely Christian, Bible-based approach, which I felt would have prevented many of the people who'd written to me from feeling comfortable enough to start recovery there. *I* couldn't have gotten better at a fervently Christian treatment center myself. Being able to pick myself up slowly but surely, and edge myself in the direction of a Higher Power, without being forced to adopt a belief system I wasn't ready for, had been part of the key to my success.

I reminded the owners that my approach had been explicitly detailed in the book, and anyone who contacted me for treatment advice after reading it probably would be looking for a place modeled after the 12-step tenets of my recovery group. I'd flown home dispirited, wishing I'd found a way to boost our meager income while also remaining involved in the eating disorder world. But endorsing this center would have been a philosophical sell-out for me, and also would have been a drastic change from everything I'd said or written about eating disorder recovery for years.

Later that week, after I'd arrived home, something happened to further convince me that aligning myself with the center would have been a huge mistake. An oversized padded envelope arrived from the center, filled with fifteen greeting cards from the eating disorder victims I'd spent time with while there, none of whom had had a week of recovery to their names. I had patiently answered all of their questions and encouraged them to be hopeful about their futures, hugging each one as I'd left.

My reward had been a condescending and judgmental packet of letters from the center's clients, sent along by the management, letting me know that they were all praying for me because I obviously didn't have the recovery I said I had. Their reasoning? I was thin and I hadn't eaten lunch at the same time they had eaten lunch, leading them to conclude that I was still binging and purging. They were praying for me, they added, to find Jesus so that I could get the help I needed.

No one writing these notes had thought to wonder if maybe I'd eaten lunch later, because I'd remained on an east coast time zone meal plan while doing my whirlwind tour. Nor had they allowed themselves to think that a woman might be thin AND in recovery—that these were not mutually exclusive concepts. The narrow-mindedness of their thinking, and the skepticism that I couldn't be in recovery because I wasn't fat, or that I didn't meet their idea of what recovery ought to look like, had enraged me.

This incident had also underscored for me that recovery really doesn't have a specific "look." Some people like me got into recovery and became thinner, partly because we weren't eating tens of thousands of calories every day anymore, and our genetic set point for weight was a little lower than other people. Some people gained a little weight, and were happier and healthier at their new weight. But whatever we all did and looked like as we settled into our healthy new bodies was appropriate, especially if we were walking the walk, and talking the talk, every day. Which I was.

Now I was sitting with a psychiatrist who had just openly told me that he wasn't sure how to know whether or not I was in recovery, based partly on what my body looked like. Was this going to follow me for the rest of my life?

"I guess you just can't know," I admitted. "You'll have to take my word for it and trust that I'm telling the truth. Why does it matter so much to you, though? How does this connect with how to deal with the Prozac debacle?"

"It matters because I'd like to put you on Wellbutrin. It acts on the dopamine pathways and not on the serotonin, and I suspect it might be a better fit for your body."

"And?" I still didn't get it.

"This medication has a side-effect of causing seizures among some bulimics who are still binging and purging. So if I put you on this drug, and you are not telling the truth about whether or not you are in recovery, there could be some very serious consequences."

He didn't have to tell me that seizures had serious consequences. I'd already lived through years of watching my husband have *seizures* while I was in my formative early years of recovery. Haywood had been rushed to the hospital by paramedics after I'd found him thrashing about in a bathroom one morning, surrounded by broken glass and medicine vials. We'd discovered that he had secondary epilepsy, and he was now on medication that controlled those seizures. I certainly wasn't going to put myself in danger of going through what I'd already witnessed.

"I am the last person who would ever lie to you about bulimia if it meant that I might have seizures," I reassured Dr. Brown. "But I cannot prove to you that I am not an active bulimic, and all you have is my word that I'm in recovery. So I'm asking you to just trust me and let me try Wellbutrin, if you think it's the right thing for me to do."

Dr. Brown looked at me. "Okay, I trust you. Let's give it a go." He scribbled another prescription and handed me my second Willy Wonka ticket to potential happiness. "But let me know how you're doing within the week," he said. "We don't want you back in the hospital."

As I left Dr. Brown's office, I was struck by this latest development in my ongoing story of recovery. Instead of being close-minded about trying an anti-depressant, I had now matured into the view that it could help me, at least temporarily. I had also continued to mature in my view of what recovery meant to me. For years, I'd felt that recovery meant eating three meals a day without purging. Now I believed that my recovery was incomplete unless I'd learned how to be more resilient and joyful, and that now included using anti-depressants, if they might help. The lack of binging and purging was still important, but it was now just a piece of the important tapestry I was weaving.

I started that day on the lowest possible dose of Wellbutrin. Over the next few days I increased the amount to what I was supposed to take, and waited. I didn't have any side-effects around fatigue this time; in fact, I had the opposite. I had been told it was a stimulant, and it definitely had that impact. I found myself awake later at night, but not to the point where I was struggling with insomnia.

I felt the full effect one magical night about two weeks later. Haywood and I had driven to a dinner in Baltimore where we were going to join some of his old lacrosse friends. We were in the restaurant when I suddenly experienced a flash of unmistakable joy. I looked down at my dress. It was red, but it suddenly looked more vividly tomato-red than it had ever looked before.

I glanced around the room, which was filled with dozens of diners, talking and enjoying their meals. But instead of just experiencing a familiar low-level buzzing of voices, I suddenly heard them as music, with everything blending into a symphonic whole. Even the sounds of forks and spoons clanking on plates and coffee cups was music to me.

My tablemates were laughing and talking about shared high school and college experiences. I felt the warmth of these friendships wash over me; I had met Haywood's friends when we were dating ten years earlier, and although I didn't know everyone well, we were all enjoying each other's company. I didn't feel inadequate, poor or stupid tonight.

In fact, I noticed, I just felt like Caroline. Flawed, imperfect Caroline, who was trying to learn how to love herself more fully and who wasn't going to stop trying until she got this happiness thing right. The Caroline who was blessed to have a husband who loved her and a son she treasured. The Caroline who had failed at one business venture, but who had gotten up off the ground again, moved forward, and gotten a new book contract. The Caroline who had fought so hard to recover from an eating disorder, and whose account of that journey had already helped thousands of other people find hope and healing. That Caroline. The one who now felt alive again, whose body was working properly, and who was back in the game of life.

If the "Right Way!" neon sign had ever flashed brightly inside me before, it was now pulsating in the happiest and most effervescent light I'd ever experienced. I was on the right road, and I was going to be okay.

## CHAPTER ELEVEN
## TRICK OR TREAT

It was Halloween night, and I was feeling more powerful, contented, and focused than I had in years. Eager to have Haywood start his Halloween tradition in a large, child-friendly neighborhood, we decided to call my parents to see if he could trick-or-treat on the same streets that Anne and I had frequented 20 years earlier. Haywood's office was very close to where I'd grown up, so it worked out perfectly.

The work that Kathleen and I had been doing together was designed to help me process and heal in new ways, but I wasn't prepared to share any of it with my parents. Blaming them for things that had happened decades ago wasn't going to change anything, so I was working on learning how to take care of myself whenever I felt triggered by their words or behaviors instead of being angry or turning inward.

One known trigger for me, however, was simply being in the house where my bulimia had been born, so I'd talked to Kathleen about how to handle Halloween without allowing an upsetting memory to mar the night.

"Just remember that this is about making sure that your son has a wonderful evening," she said. "If you feel triggered by being in the house, or your parents make a comment about your appearance, you have the emotional tools to walk away without engaging. Remember that you are an adult and not a child any longer. Leave, take deep breaths, change the subject, or laugh. But don't engage with them."

Still, driving the familiar road to my house took me back in time. I passed grocery stores where I had once shoplifted food and laxatives and passed through neighborhoods that reminded me of difficult times in my life. As I saw the spires of the National Cathedral in the distance, I thought back to my four years of bulimia there, and wished that I could have been a different person. I'd always loved school, but with a part-time job like bulimia, being fully enthralled with learning had been pretty difficult.

I had mixed feelings as I drove up to my old house. My parents loved my son, so I knew that he'd be a distraction from talking about anything else, but my stomach still churned uneasily whenever I came home. I would have preferred to stay away completely as I went through therapy, but my grandmother, Donny, had now moved into my parents' home, and I wanted to see her as often I could.

I went in through the back gate, my green dragon behind me. He still didn't really comprehend this holiday, so we'd have to walk him through his first few houses, and explain that you could get a bunch of candy if you just rang a doorbell and said, "Trick or Treat!" Learning you could get something for nothing was going to be a magic moment for Haywood, as it is for every child.

I left Haywood in the kitchen with my parents while I bounded up the stairs to see Donny, who was now living in my old bedroom. My grandmother's attitude toward life had always been playful, childlike, and intelligent, plus she had pulled off something I found amazing: although she had three grandchildren whom she adored equally, we *all* thought we were her favorite.

"Donny!" I threw my arms around her.

"Eence Teence Weence!" she exclaimed happily, using her old nickname for me. "Why are you here?"

"It's Halloween, Donny. We brought Haywood here so that he could learn how to trick or treat like I used to. Remember when Anne and I would go out on Halloween together?"

I loved to reminisce with Donny. She had been like another grandmother to Anne, just as hers had been to me.

"Oh, yes. How could I forget? You won't stay out late with Haywood will you? You and Anne were always out so late," she noted disapprovingly. It was like I was still nine to her, and it felt nice to know that her concerns had always come from love.

"No, we're just going to do a few houses because we have to drive back tonight."

At that moment, we heard my husband's booming voice from downstairs shout, "Trick or Treat!" Haywood had known this house for over ten years, and he was often greeted more warmly here than I was. Once, my father had even noted that I'd "taken Haywood down in the world" because I'd brought my bulimia into the marriage as a secret partner. Haywood had mixed feelings about how to treat my parents; while he hated some of the things he'd heard from me and already observed, he tried to have a cordial relationship with them for the sake of our child. In fact, we were both on a tightrope.

"Let's go C," Haywood yelled from the bottom of the stairs. "It's getting dark."

I stood up to give Donny another hug and glanced at the familiar desk where I'd done thousands of hours of homework to get through National Cathedral School and into Harvard. Out of the corner of my eye, I saw the mirror where I had stood and hated my body so viciously and violently. Donny was sleeping in the same bed where I'd spent many miserable nights after binges and purges, or fights with my parents. The bathroom where I had swallowed syrup of ipecac to induce episodes of awful vomiting was just steps away. Right below, where my son now was waiting for me, was where I'd been derisively called "the bad seed." Suddenly, even though I loved my grandmother, I couldn't wait to get out of there.

"I'll see you soon Donny," I promised, giving her a long hug and kiss as I got up to leave.

Passing the mirror, I adjusted my gold jacket. I was wearing a form-fitting cat suit that left nothing to the imagination. I was even wearing a suede belt over my stomach, which I never would have done five years earlier while I was fighting to love my body. Now I didn't hesitate to buy a tight outfit and wear a belt—something that had silently taunted me after binges when I was bloated and my stomach hurt to the touch.

I turned sideways and glanced at my profile. I looked normal, but something felt wrong. I adjusted the belt and wondered why I was feeling odd. Maybe it was just because Dr. Brown had said that people with eating disorder histories are exquisitely sensitive to any changes to their bodies, and I was getting a touch of the flu. That had to be it.

I turned away from the mirror and clattered down the stairs, where I heard Haywood explaining to our son how Halloween works.

"You take this bucket and go up to people's doors and ring their doorbell," he began. "Then, when they open the door, you shout, 'Trick-or-treat!' and they put candy in your bucket."

My son's eyes widened as he grasped the excitement of Halloween's "something for nothing" bargain.

"Do you think you can do that?"

"I do it!" Haywood screamed, eagerly darting out the door.

* * * * * * * *

IN THE DAYS following Halloween, I continued to feel strange. I didn't know what was going on, but I figured it was a minor flu and would pass. It was interesting to notice during this period that Haywood's bag of Halloween candy lay in our kitchen untouched by me. I felt no urge to reach in and help myself to any of my old binge foods, including Three Musketeers, Milky Ways and Sugar Mamas. Although I'd been in recovery for many years, I hadn't lived anywhere since 1984 where a tempting bag of candy was lying around unguarded. I was delighted to note that despite being alone much of the day with the candy one room away from where I was writing, I simply didn't eat it, want it, or feel tempted to sneak a piece to "get away" with it. There was no one I needed to fool or hide from anymore; my respect for myself was all that mattered.

Within the week, I was showering when I noticed that my breasts felt more tender than normal. The pieces tumbled into place. *I had to be pregnant.* There was no other explanation, and it all made sense now. Within an hour I had gotten a pregnancy test and my answer: I was expecting a baby.

Unlike the joy I'd felt when I discovered I was expecting Haywood, I now felt nothing but dread. Haywood and I had decided that we had to be on more solid financial footing and in a larger house before we had another child, so I was using birth control. Clearly, it hadn't worked.

Another thought filled my mind with fear. I went to the bathroom and found the bottle with my Wellbutrin prescription. With trembling fingers, I called information to get the number for the pharmaceutical company's headquarters.

"May I speak with your director of publicity?" I asked when I reached the company. I didn't know where else to start, and as a former publicist, I thought that the person would at least know who else I needed to talk to if they didn't have the answers I needed.

A pleasant-sounding man was connected with me. "How may I help you?"

"Hi, I've been on Wellbutrin for a little while and I just found out I'm pregnant. Do you have any idea if there have been studies done on the impact of this drug on a fetus?"

"There have been no studies done," he responded efficiently. "There have been some studies done on Prozac and pregnancy, but that's all I can tell you. Prozac works on a different chemical pathway, though, so I'm not even sure if those studies would be helpful to you."

Great. I thanked him and hung up. Dr. Brown had told me not to get pregnant while I was on Wellbutrin because he wanted my moods to stabilize and for me to have a period of hormonal and chemical stability before I added the stress of another child. I had assured him that we had no plans to have another child, and I had meant it.

Now this. I adored my son and wanted another child but I didn't want one *now*.

Shit. What was I going to do? The thought of an abortion crossed my mind. If the baby was deformed, I'd never forgive myself. A number of friends and classmates over the years had had abortions, and for most of them it had been no big deal, or so they'd told me.

I gazed at the historic South Mountain from my desk. It was a gorgeous fall day, with the reds, auburn and gold colors lighting up the slopes. A clock tower on Middletown's main street, dating from the early 1800s, chimed 10 am in the distance. I sat there, staring out the window, thinking about the craziness of my life. Why did I have a pattern of upending stability with life-changing jolts like this? Every time I had a placid moment—Boom!—a bomb went off, and I had to scramble for cover and figure out how to survive.

But maybe that was the lesson—that life really is nothing but a series of jolts and setbacks, followed by resilience and positive growth. And that recovery from my eating disorder was going to be a series of challenges that I'd need to overcome, one at a time, without using food as a way to cope.

I closed my eyes. There was a child growing inside me. I could even feel it. Images of Haywood's birth, the joy he'd brought us, and how being a mother had helped me to become a better person filled my head.

But was it the right time to go through this again? And what if the baby was irreparably harmed because I'd taken pills to boost my happiness? As these questions coursed in an endless loop through my head, they were answered by a surprising part of my consciousness: "There's never a 'right' time for anything, Caroline," I heard. "Who are you to play God?"

My eyes snapped open. I looked around. I was alone. But it FELT like someone was talking to me.

The voice had gotten my attention, though. It was true. There was no perfect time for anything, and left to our decisions, Haywood and I might never feel like we had enough money to have another baby. And what was "enough money," anyway? We were raising one child now with a little money and lots of debt. We could do it again, if we had to.

Many minutes ticked by as I thought about every possibility. There was so much to consider: money, the impact of Wellbutrin, our cramped living situation. I was too flooded to decide on my own, so I closed my eyes to pray for guidance, much as I once had when I'd been at my wits' end in early recovery, uncertain of whether or not I had what it took to get better.

"God, I know you're out there, and that you're always waiting for me to ask questions so that I can listen for your answers, and I really need your help today," I began. "I'm pregnant and I really don't know if it's selfish to continue a pregnancy that might not be healthy, and I'm really confused. I love being a mother, but I wasn't thinking that this was the right time to have another baby, so I need to know what to do. Please send me a sign and tell me what to do. Please. Amen."

I waited, but nothing happened. No lights, voices or noises from beyond interrupted my quiet. Instead, I gradually felt the peace that always descended on me whenever I stopped struggling and the correct answer entered my consciousness. My ever-trusty internal neon sign start to pulse "Right way!" along with a certain feeling that whatever unfolded was going to be part of a divine plan that was already at work.

I knew what I had to do. I put my hand protectively over my stomach and picked up the phone to call Haywood at work. I had to tell him that he was going to be a Daddy again. Then I had to prepare myself to deal with my life, which had just gone topsy-turvy again.

# CHAPTER TWELVE
## THE WORKING MOM

As I'd suspected, Haywood was initially taken aback at the prospect of a second child, particularly in light of the small house and the fact that we were just getting back on our feet financially. But he quickly warmed up to the idea of being a dad again, so we had a small celebration that night in honor of the unborn baby who would join us during the following summer, probably smack in the middle of the 1992 Atlanta Olympic Games.

Pictures from that time in our lives show us looking happy and healthy, which was mostly true. Haywood's company was going like gangbusters, and through a series of skillful acquisitions and management, the company's stock options were becoming more and more valuable by the day, which made us feel increasingly hopeful about our financial prospects, despite the sky-high debt. In addition to making steady progress on my new book, *Feeding the Soul*, I was also being courted for a marketing job that might pay well, and that would allow me to help people find quality eating disorder treatment while mostly continuing to work from home.

A large hospital chain, seeing the rise in addiction treatment services, had decided to jump in with both feet and open a freestanding women's unit devoted to eating disorders and depression in one of their Midwest hospitals. The idea they were pitching to me was that I would help them design the program, advise them on publicity, and be the "face" of the organization in exchange for a flexible job that could pick up where Renewal left off. It felt like this surprising and timely offer might be God's consolation prize for Renewal being such a bust. Perhaps, I mused, this position would allow me to serve the field in a meaningful way, fulfilling my original desire while also allowing me to be a flexible working mom who could work from home. It sounded almost too good to be true.

The developments around my body were another story. It was ironic that I'd been recently congratulating myself on my ability to stay within my comfortable eating guidelines, despite having a bag of candy in the house with me all day. Within two weeks of finding out I was pregnant, food was the enemy all over again—but not from a bulimic standpoint. The morning sickness I'd experienced with my first pregnancy hit full-force again, complete with the all-day nausea and nasty metallic taste in my mouth from the moment I awoke to the moment I went to bed. Grocery shopping, the skill I'd grown so proud of in recovery, was now snatched away again, despite my best efforts to force myself into this environment.

"Mommy! What wrong?" my two-year-old son would exclaim with a sad face as I entered grocery stores with him. Like a vampire spotting its first ray of sunshine, the glimpse of a produce section would cause me to shudder and flee its disgusting sights and smells, despite every good intention to soldier through the task of buying and preparing food for our family.

"Mrs. Miller, as I told you before, morning sickness is the sign of a very healthy pregnancy," my doctor informed me in an effort to allay my fears about Wellbutrin on the developing fetus. Nothing he said, though, removed the lurking fear that I might have unwittingly hurt my baby. I knew this would be a worry I would have until I delivered in July, so I just hunkered down to wait out the morning sickness and whatever else might happen over the coming months. After giving birth to one child and going bankrupt almost immediately after that event, I was starting to feel like having children might be the harbinger of bad news that would ultimately make me stronger in some way. Maybe this one would be no different.

Because of my frequent bouts in bed with fatigue and nausea, I put off my in-person interview with the hospital chain as long as possible. I negotiated the details of the job by phone, and only agreed to meet face-to-face toward the end of my first trimester when my face didn't look so pinched and ashen. Just before Christmas 1991, I dressed as professionally as I could, firmly buttoning a black blazer over my bulging stomach. I was showing signs of a child much sooner than I had the first time around, which I was unprepared for. I didn't think it would be a good idea to advertise my condition.

Jill Richards was on a multi-state swing, and was touching down in Baltimore briefly just to interview me. We had agreed to meet at the airport, about an hour from my home. I parked and found the restaurant where we had arranged to meet.

At the appointed moment, I felt Jill coming my way before I actually recognized her from the description she'd provided. Her energy, which vibrated over the phone lines, was no less apparent as she clicked towards the booth where I waited.

"You must be Caroline!" she announced loudly. "So nice to meet you!"

I couldn't help but notice that Jill was impeccably groomed from the tip of her brunette bob to the points of her fashionable shoes. Her nails and heels were scarlet. They matched. I protectively curled my fingers into a fist so that she wouldn't see my bitten-to-the-quick nails and I suddenly wondered if anything I was wearing matched. I felt old and frumpy.

I rose and tried to suck in my stomach. "So nice to meet you, too, after all these weeks," I responded. "You look as pulled-together as you sound on the phone!" Although I was rarely intimidated, I suddenly felt like I wasn't of the same caliber as this fast-talking, sharp New Yorker, even though she hadn't said anything that would lead me to believe she felt that way about me. (I made a mental note to talk to Kathleen about my initial pessimistic reaction.)

Jill didn't waste any time as soon as we were done with pleasantries. She only had an hour between flights, and kept glancing at her watch to make sure that we kept the conversation moving on the right track.

"As you know, we want you to come to Kansas City once a month or so to help us design and implement a program for women with dual diagnoses—eating disorders and depression," Jill rapidly explained. "Your job would also include giving speeches, being in our advertising, and responding to all media queries. We would also like you to help us drum up clients for this wing, many of whom might be interested in our unit because of your book."

The job sounded doable and straightforward. No surprises from what we'd talked about. As she'd already said on the phone, I would be able to work from home for the most part; my trips to Kansas City would be no more than 48 hours in length, and would occur about once a month. It appeared that I could write marketing brochures, help the program director design a protocol for eating disorder treatment, and do everything from the comfort of Middletown in my pajamas. The unit's opening date was a month before the baby's due date, which was also perfect for me.

I mentioned that I was grateful for the flexibility of the job, particularly in light of my son being only 2 years old. I wasn't completely past the miscarriage point for my current pregnancy, so I didn't want to say that I was expecting unless I was directly asked. I wasn't. So I confirmed the piece of the job that mattered the most to me: "Are you sure that I don't have to travel much?"

"Nope. We want your guidance and experience in the field as we dip our toe into this area," Jill answered. "If it's profitable, we'd like to talk to you about doing more work with us on future projects, and the time commitment and travel might change at that point."

I was curious. "Do you travel a lot?" Jill looked so sleek and competent that I wondered how she managed to do what she did, particularly if she was on the road often. I found that doing anything for myself like getting dressed, with a hyperactive two-year-old anywhere nearby, took me twice as long as it had before. I would also frequently discover later that in the rush to pack a diaper bag with books, food and other toddler essentials, I'd leave something—maybe one earring off. Jill looked like she never forgot earrings, and that not only did she probably always have two of them, they undoubtedly matched her handbag, shoes, or anything else that had hardware.

"I travel about three to four days a week," she replied. "I love it. We have hospitals in a lot of states, and I need to oversee all of them because their marketing directors answer to me. We count how many beds are full in our facilities every Friday, and that's how we determine whether or not my efforts and people are being successful. It keeps me hopping." She looked down at her discreet gold watch again to subtly underscore her point.

"I hope you don't mind my asking... do you have children?"

Jill smiled her first genuine smile, and her eyes softened. "Two. They're great—8 and 10."

"Is it tough to balance juggling work and travel with two small kids?"

"No, not really," she answered, pulling pictures out of her purse to show me. The children were adorable.

Jill continued her answer after putting the pictures away. "I have a full-time nanny who has been with us since the kids were born, and they call her 'Mom.' They call me 'Mommy,' isn't that cute? I don't know what I'd do without her. And my husband is home every night, so it works really well. I'm home on the weekends, and the kids just expect that I'm gone from Monday through Thursday—no big deal."

I studied her face. I didn't think she was making it up. I could identify with the fleeting enjoyment of having some time away from the house to pursue something that was important to me, but I couldn't make the mental leap of being away the bulk of the week without touching, smelling, or playing with my children.

But it was clear that being a working mother had many definitions. While a lot of travel worked for some, it was probably never going to be the way I made a living. If I was going to be the happy and fulfilled mom I wanted to be, I would have to cobble together a variety of types of work that would allow me enough flexibility to earn money and still put my children's needs first whenever necessary. The job I was being offered would be a good taste of a certain type of commuting lifestyle with flexibility. I decided to go for it.

"So we have a deal?" Jill stood and closed our meeting with a cold, firm handshake. "You'll be the assistant director of marketing for the Kansas City unit, and then we'll look around for another one for you to work on if this one goes well." She pulled a contract out of her briefcase, which had information on healthcare benefits and other company perks, and told me to go through the documents carefully and call with any questions.

"Sounds great!" I shook her hand with enthusiasm and drove back to Middletown as a professionally-employed, corporate woman, with a salary, benefits and a possible future in the healthcare field. Life, I thought, was really going our way again. God was good.

\* \* \* \* \* \* \* \*

Kathleen and I had agreed to add group therapy to my weekly regimen in the months preceding my new pregnancy. Our work had progressed to the point where I was ready to experience the unvarnished feedback of new people and to be vulnerable with others about my self-doubts. The difference between this and my prior self-help eating disorder support group was that the group was overseen by Kathleen and her professional colleague, Carole. If I overreacted or became defensive with someone, I could address it and work through it immediately with their guidance. It was also a chance for me to hear about the concerns and dreams of new men and women, and to learn from them as they wrestled with their own challenges and personal issues.

I had always had the opinion that therapy wasn't for sissies, ever since my first bout with it in 1984 when I was starting my bulimia recovery. In the hands of the right professional, the digging and introspective work was exceptionally challenging, but it had a huge payoff. However difficult I'd found individual therapy to be, group therapy trumped it by far. On a number of occasions as I'd revealed feelings of shame or episodes of childish behavior, I'd dug my fingernails into the soft arm cushions to prevent me from fleeing before I bore the full brunt of being "seen" by others. Although I did have a number of difficult evenings in that office, where I'd been accurately confronted about some of my misperceptions of others' intentions, I'd also found that these near-strangers offered me healing and acceptance in uncharted ways.

Despite the challenges of opening myself up to being observed and judged by my peers as trained mental health professionals observed, I loved group therapy. I was mesmerized by watching other people bare their souls and fears and then receive both positive and critical feedback. If scabs were ripped off some old emotional wound here, the person had to sit with the pain publicly and then work through it in front of us. In my eating disorder group, on the other hand, all feelings were processed alone or with our peers afterwards, and without professional guidance. Both of these modalities had their benefits, I had decided, and both had been enormously helpful in different ways at different moments in my life. My free support group had given me the courage to be honest and share. Individual therapy had given me a safe environment to start my inner healing. Now group therapy was taking me to deeper and more exposed places. They had built on each other, and every step had been essential in my journey.

The group was a stalwart support for me over several months as I continued to chip away at my occasional guilt around leaving my son in daycare, being pregnant again under less-than-ideal circumstances, and integrating some of my childhood memories with adult insights around feeling worthy. They'd laughed and cried with me, and I'd also been privileged to watch some of these brave people deal with issues ranging from the pain of working with dying children to receiving medical death sentences themselves.

I wasn't the only person who wasn't always sure about how to bond with others and develop rewarding friendships. I learned as I watched mature men and women openly admit to feelings of insecurity and fear about being in any kind of relationship, followed by Kathleen and Ronnie's pushing and probing for deeper meaning and personal connections. In this protected environment, we all felt free to say whatever came to mind, no matter how crazy it sounded. I lost count of how often people exclaimed, "You feel that way, too? I thought I was the only person who thought like that!"

Although I'd watched and participated in some of the verbal sparring that arose whenever one of us was irritated by someone else's behavior, I'd never been the target of another person's direct anger. That all changed one balmy spring evening as I sat in my customary chair near the door, hands folded protectively over the bump under my sundress.

It was my turn to talk about how my week had gone, and I felt relaxed and positive as I discussed the developments around my monthly travel, our finances, and my comfort with my expanding body and new food choices.

"I'm feeling good tonight," I opened. "I'm in my seventh year of recovery from my eating disorder, and I'm grateful that I have a body that can even get pregnant again. I'm past the morning sickness and I'm handling the food cravings and weight gain well. I'm doing the same 'turn around on the scale and plug your ears' thing with the doctor for my Ob/Gyn visits, and it works for me. I'm also liking my job with the hospital chain, and I think I'm doing well with their marketing and planning. All in all, no complaints. I'm in an okay place and I'm happy about that."

I was about to continue with some other upbeat thoughts when Kristen, a bulky redhead across the room, announced that she was angry and needed to say something important.

Startled by the interruption, I immediately stopped talking and looked at her. Seven men and women, and two therapists, also turned expectantly in her direction.

"I'm feeling resentful right now," she began. "Caroline has the perfect life—she's pretty, blonde, a Harvard graduate, and she's married to a Harvard guy, too. It's like Barbie and Ken on top of the wedding cake, or something like that, and everything seems to go her way. I don't want to hear about her eating disorder anymore, either, because she's even thin despite being pregnant. In my opinion, it's not such a bad thing to have gone through an eating disorder if you end up looking like that. I've even been thinking about trying to throw up occasionally because I could stand to lose a few pounds myself."

No one knew what to say. We let her words just hang in the room, unanswered. The silence felt incredibly loud.

Kathleen finally intervened. "Do you think it's possible that your anger has nothing to do with Caroline at all? Do you really think that her life, and her eating disorder recovery, has been without struggle? Do you have any compassion for her and what she has shared here with us about what she's had to do to even sit here and be pregnant?"

Kristen was silent for a moment, her red face matching the crimson flush that was rising on her ample chest. She was a teacher in the local school system, and I knew from listening to her for many months that she struggled with her own feelings of inadequacy around her weight, her multiple failed relationships, and her concern that she wasn't pursuing a profession that brought her more joy than frustration. I had offered my own words of support on many occasions, and I'd thought that we had developed a tentative friendship of sorts, with mutual respect. I wondered now if that had all been one-way.

Kristen finally spoke. "Caroline reminds me of my brother. He was good-looking and he always got everything he wanted—girls, good grades, good jobs, you name it. No struggles, my parents adored him, and everything looked effortless. When I look at Caroline, I see the same thing—no struggle, no worries, good looks and good grades. She's him."

Again, we were all quiet. Kristen and the entire group knew a fair amount about my history, none of which included an easy walk through the park. My company's bankruptcy had been discussed here, along with painful stories about my childhood and feelings of abandonment by my parents. But Kristen had clearly not registered much of it, and instead was reacting to me tonight as if I was a billboard. I was just a fetching picture with nothing behind me—no depth, challenge or interest. I would forever be a four-part visual sound bite to her: thin, blond, pretty and Harvard grad, with any one of those four facts being enough to trigger resentment.

The rest of the group leapt to my defense, which felt good. It also surprised me. I had often felt alone throughout my early and teen years, accustomed to not having anyone show up at my side if I needed it. The "bad seed" memory flitted through my head.

"Are you crazy?" Bob said. "Don't you remember how she lost her house and had to move into that monster mansion in bankruptcy? That doesn't count as a struggle in your book?"

Kira spoke next. "You want to try bulimia because she's thin now? Didn't you hear her say that she was heavy and bloated during her eating disorder years, and that she doesn't even want to weigh herself during pregnancy because she's been stable at a comfortable weight for years because she doesn't know the numbers? Do you think she's thin because she used to throw up? Are you kidding? You want to put yourself through years of hell because you think it would help you lose weight? Did you consider that she might be thin because it's her set point and she takes care of herself after years of not doing it?"

I stayed quiet for the most part as Kristen gradually acknowledged that her reaction to me was misplaced fury about how her parents had never recognized her own unique gifts and efforts, but had instead focused on the ease with which her brother had mastered so many things in life. She'd never felt validated or loved by them, she admitted, and something about what I had presented tonight had caused her to erupt. If I'd been in a business setting, and someone had gotten angry because I triggered something similar in them, I never would have had the benefit of understanding what was behind their emotions, and would have probably blamed myself for any sour feelings that arose. Through group therapy, though, I was really learning more about how I appeared to others, for better or for worse, and what assumptions I also made about other people that were either accurate or unfounded. That skill, I later discovered, showed up later at a time when I couldn't have needed it more.

## CHAPTER THIRTEEN
## GETTING CLOSURE ON THE FIRST THIRTY

Middletown had always felt the way it sounded: we were in the middle, going from one place to the other; it wasn't our final destination. Most of our boxes remained in the unfinished concrete basement of the small house, untouched since the day we'd moved in. While we had enjoyed our neighbors, they were all much older and we never went beyond being outsiders who had plopped down in the middle of their street, with no roots or anchors in the local society.

So it was with a sense of relief and excitement that Haywood and I got word that the tenant in our condominium in Baltimore was ready to move out, which coincided perfectly with the end of our one-year lease in the Middletown house. I was in my fifth month of pregnancy, starting to feel ungainly, so relocating to our old, familiar Charm City locale couldn't have come at a better time. When we'd moved out of the city so that we could experience the aloneness and isolation of our Boring farmette, being with people hadn't been a priority. We'd wanted a peaceful place to plan our lives and unwind at the end of the day.

Now, we couldn't wait to return to the streets where I'd first found my recovery, where Haywood had been born, and where we knew so many people who cared about us. I'd had enough of loneliness (no social gatherings, unless group therapy counted) and quiet days. I'd never again underestimate the power of being connected, particularly in person with other people. This was a powerful lesson in my wanderings from Boring to Middletown and now back to Baltimore—other people mattered. Happiness isn't really possible without those meaningful bonds.

In March of 1992, a Mayflower moving van pulled up to our Middletown house and filled up. I could barely contain myself. My only sadness was that our two dogs had to find good homes because the condo wouldn't accept them. As a going away gift to Sherri, who had been a warm and fun presence in my son's life every day for over a year, we gave her our black Labrador mutt, Ajax, who needed room to run and cows to bark at. Haywood didn't know that we were saying goodbye for the last time, but I did as we pulled away from Sherri's farm. This wonderful family daycare setting, which had once felt like an admission of maternal failure, had been nothing but positive for me and my son—another powerful learning experience for which I was grateful.

Desdemona, an Australian shepherd mix, went to Annapolis to live with a family that had three children who desperately wanted a pet. Desi, as we called her, was a lover, and she was particularly comforting to their middle child, whose birth deformities as a result of being a preemie had left her partially blind. Although I hated parting with our pets, especially on top of giving away our horses when we'd moved to Middletown in a rush, I was at least relieved that both dogs had happy places to live.

Settling back into Baltimore felt like putting on warm slippers. I immediately reconnected with my eating disorder support group meetings and reveled in the familiar friendships. I marveled as I walked into the comforting self-help evening meetings with my needlepoint canvases, remembering that I'd once sat in these church basements and college classrooms with a feeling of desperation and hope, not even sure I could have children. Now, eight years later, I was an "old-timer" who offered hope to the people who reminded me so much of the person I'd once been, now with one successful pregnancy behind me and another one underway. One day at a time, regardless of what was going on around me, I'd pulled the rabbit out of the hat. I was in recovery and nothing had shaken me from that place.

My work with the hospital chain was going according to plan. Once my stomach had gotten too large to hide, I'd told Jill that I had a baby coming in July, weeks after the planned opening of the unit. I detected a flicker of disappointment in her voice when I called her with the news. I wanted to tell her that I'd been surprised by the pregnancy too, and that birth control clearly was fallible, but we didn't have the kind of relationship that would allow me to be so intimate. I also wanted to give her notice that if we agreed to continue to work together after the unit's opening, I'd need at least two months with my baby before I was ready to work again. Again, I detected disappointment in her voice. Had I just said something wrong? Something told me that Jill probably hadn't taken off two months after having her two kids. Whoops.

No one ever complained about my work ethic or performance on the hospital unit, though. I wanted my efforts to speak for me, and they did. I transferred all of the energy I'd once had for Renewal into lavishing time and thought on the design of the hospital unit. The occasional trips to Kansas City turned out to be fun. Although I was nearly thirty, I'd never traveled much on my own, so navigating rental car counters and getting myself to and from airports helped me feel more self-sufficient. I often thought to myself that although I was behind the curve on professional habits, I was probably ahead of most of my peers in terms of self-reflection due to an addiction, and learning about my own resilience. Falling apart in my twenties, on every front, had had a silver lining.

* * * * * * * *

ONE OF THE MOST important things I had to do after we moved back to Baltimore, was to get a sonogram to check on the baby's progress. It was a few weeks later than I'd had one for our first child, so I expected to hear that I had a large baby again. I wasn't ready for what the sonogram technician told me as I lay on the uncomfortable gurney, a cold stethoscope sliding over the slimy goo on my belly.

The tech measured something on the screen once, and then twice, and turned to me. "Those are the biggest feet I've ever seen on a fetus at this stage of a pregnancy," he said in surprise.

"What?" I sat up abruptly. "How can you tell?"

"Here." He quickly manipulated the image on the screen and jabbed some buttons. "There are the baby's feet, see? Those are some flippers!" He zoomed his cold scope around on my belly a bit more, explaining, "Here's the head, there's the elbow, there's the heart, there's the spine…" It all looked like a black and white alien to me, but I didn't hear that anything looked amiss or deformed. I breathed out and lay back down. Big feet would not be a problem.

"Want to know what you're having?" The tech looked at me. I hadn't expected this. We hadn't known the sex of our first baby, and I'd loved the surprise of hearing "It's a boy!" as my son made his debut. But I suddenly wanted to know what was growing inside of me. After years of occasionally not knowing where we'd live, or how we'd earn our next dime, having concrete information appealed to me.

"Yes. Tell me what I'm having." I felt like I was about to get a Christmas present. I knew I'd be happy with either a boy or a girl, so any news would be good.

"It's a girl!" He smiled at me. "And it looks like she's gonna be a big one!"

Although I was delighted to hear that Haywood was going to have a sister, something about the way the tech announced my daughter's presence, and her size, made me careen back to my childhood, when I'd heard "You're so big!" over and over again. There was no question that being told I was "big" in every situation, from the time I was old enough to understand that I was being described in a way that didn't fit everyone else's bodies, had played a role in formulating my perception of myself as "fat." Although no one had actually *said* I was "fat," my brain had heard it that way, and without group therapy for tots, I hadn't been able to explore whether or not I actually was overweight. The domino effect had been to inch me towards hating my body, followed by the bulimia.

I didn't want my daughter ever to feel the same confusion I'd felt about what "big" meant, now that I had an inkling that she might, indeed, be a tall girl, too—with "flippers." It didn't sound particularly attractive, and I walked out of the medical office with a fresh goal that I hadn't had when I walked in.

I was going to give birth to a daughter, and the greatest gift I could give her would be to raise her with a feeling of pride in her body and the self-esteem I'd never had. I was still a work in progress myself, but I was deadly serious about what I knew lay ahead of me. I was bringing a daughter into a world that still expected women to be pretty and thin, and getting her through the storms of puberty without having her succumb to the pressures that nailed me was now one of the biggest long-term goals I'd ever set for myself. Failure was not an option.

\* \* \* \* \* \* \* \*

"WHEN ARE YOU DUE, ma'am?" The stewardess eyed my stomach ominously. I was slipping my last flight to Kansas City in just under hitting the 8th month, at which point I knew I'd have to stop flying.

"Next month—mid-July," I answered. It was early June and I was on my way to Kansas City to speak at the hospital wing's grand opening the following day. I was also scheduled to film some television advertisements for the unit, which would be shot strategically to avoid any belly angles, as well as talk to local reporters. I wasn't worried about my water breaking or delivering early because I felt fine, but a 5'10" woman with a huge stomach was definitely a sight to behold, and I had caught the stewardess's eye.

"Ma'am, we'd like you to sit in first class," she said carefully. "We'd just like to keep an eye on you, and we have some extra spaces to offer. Would that be okay?"

"Oh, that would be great. Thank you." Baltimore was in the midst of a heat wave, and spreading my swollen body out into a wider seat was a welcome idea. I sank into the leather seat and closed my eyes.

I was glad this was my last trip. Although I definitely wanted the unit to succeed, my nesting instincts had kicked in, and I'd been cleaning every surface of the condo in preparation for our daughter's arrival. A frilly pink dress with matching bonnet now hung on the mobile over the crib that was waiting for Samantha. Leaving town was getting harder and I was looking forward to having some time off.

Jill had been asking me more pointed questions about my desire to work after Samantha's birth. I had already named this little girl in my stomach after my favorite childhood show, "Bewitched," in which the main character used her magical powers to make dreams come true. My Samantha would be a good witch, too, I'd decided. On top of that, every time I'd speak her name I would be reminded of the happy hours I'd once whiled away in front of the television, entranced by the power of sorcery and make-believe.

I told Jill that I was somewhat ambivalent about returning to the working world too quickly, but that I wanted to remain open to the possibility of starting work again in the fall, depending on how well the unit was received. I had two months of paid maternity leave awaiting me, and I intended to take every minute of it. Sometimes I suspected that Jill felt I'd taken advantage of the hospital by joining them just as I'd hit my first trimester, but they'd never asked a single question about my intentions of getting pregnant when they were courting me. I would have volunteered my status if asked because telling the truth had been an ingrained part of getting well.

"You're only as sick as your secrets," I'd heard in meeting rooms again and again for years, and the fallout, many years later, is that I still reflexively tell the truth when asked a question, even if it isn't necessarily in my best interests.

The nesting instincts at home had been matched by a desired to slow down in other areas of my life. As I imagined the demands of a newborn and a three-year-old son, I realized that my evening group therapy sessions probably wouldn't be possible any longer. Kathleen and I had agreed to announce it to the group with several weeks' lead time so that we could all process my leave-taking.

On the night of my last group therapy session, we did our familiar "goodbye" ritual. I'd been through it once before with a woman who needed to leave for professional reasons, so I was prepared with tissues. We took turns going around the group as I took in their comments about my growth in the group and their hopes for my future.

Elinor was first. I'd initially been afraid of Elinor because she was a doctor who talked in short bursts, and made clinical diagnoses of all of us that sounded harsher and colder than she meant them to sound. Through the group feedback, she'd learned how to slow down and connect more thoughtfully with all of us, and she made a point of noting that she had appreciated my direct suggestions about her verbal tendencies.

"You have a good eye for what is really going on with people," she said. "Just be careful not to always share it with people who aren't ready to hear it. My concern for you is that you could be a lightning rod for criticism because you speak your mind, but I want you to know how much I've learned from you in a lot of different ways because of it. Thank you for being here, and for allowing me to see past what other people might not."

Bob was next. He was the shyest member of the group, and had always stuttered when he said something important. I was impressed by his courage in facing his stutter with us, and for pushing through it to make sure he got his messages out. He started his farewell to me by saying, "I can finally tell you how much it drove me crazy when you talked about New Age stuff!"

We all erupted in laughter because it was a big step for Bob to say that he disliked anything. The good thing about his revelation was that I didn't take offense. It was okay to be different and not feel bad, and for others to have their opinions, whether or not I agreed. I had learned that here.

Kristen cried more than I did as she bade me farewell. "I'm going to miss you, and I want you to know that I admire how far you've come. Thank you for letting me go off on you that night, and for not hating me as a result. It helped me to see how deep-seated my own angers and insecurities are around my brother, and I doubt I would have had that breakthrough unless you'd been here. Let's please stay in touch."

I read my own goodbye letters and felt like I'd done a good job of backing up my observations of others' growth with specific incidents. I told each person what I had learned from them, and what I hoped they would have in their future.

Saying goodbye to Garrett was the hardest, because he was the first openly gay person with AIDS I had ever known. He had been coming to our group to help him deal with the fact that doctors had told him he didn't have more than a year to live. Garrett was the first person with AIDS whom I had ever touched or hugged, and I thanked him for educating me not to be afraid of the disease, and to be able to express my love around it. He had also opened my eyes to the world of discrimination, painfully describing incidents in which he'd been ignored or criticized by people who were ignorant about homosexuality. Not seeing Garrett anymore, or watching his brave battle to die with grace and at peace, was going to be hard for me. I could barely finish my goodbye without breaking down completely.

"Whenever I think about my life being hard, I think about what you face every day, and I'm humbled," I concluded. "I'm honored to know you and to call you my friend."

That evening had been important closure for me; it was one of the first times I'd actually "done closure" well. I had a tendency to walk away from painful situations, like moving to Middletown without telling my program friends why, without processing the full brunt of what I was leaving behind. The group had taught me how crucial it is to end relationships with no dangling threads, and nothing left unsaid, so I had no regrets as I drove away that last night in 1992.

＊ ＊ ＊ ＊ ＊ ＊ ＊ ＊

THE OPENING OF the hospital unit went well. We cut ribbons, I gave speeches, signed books, and mingled with clients who were already on the unit as patients. All of the women who were there had a mixture of depression and an eating disorder. Some were cutters, who exorcised their inner demons through the satisfaction of feeling pain and seeing blood flow from their self-inflicted wounds. Some had suffered incest by a father or stepfather, or had been sexually abused by someone else. I talked to the patients when it was appropriate, but I had the uncomfortable feeling that I simply wasn't able to tap into or assuage their misery.

The stories I heard made me incredibly sad. Instead of shaking off the tales of childhood abuse and food addiction, I felt pulled down. What was wrong with me? Had I lost my empathy and resilience? Why wasn't I more hopeful after talking to the women, buoyed by knowing that my recovery might be a beacon of hope to them? The old fire that had driven me to share my recovery so widely, first in a book and then in the media, had died down. I needed to find out why.

When I got home to Baltimore I talked to Kathleen about my conflicting feelings about working in the eating disorder field. "It sounded and felt like the right thing to do when I was offered the job," I explained. "But I'm not sure I want to do this type of work any longer. What has happened to me?" I was truly puzzled.

"Maybe you've changed. Maybe your energies need to go somewhere else now. Maybe you are being called to another field." Because I knew Kathleen so well, I knew that I was supposed to pick up on this last sentence and speculate on what other field that might be. Nothing came to mind, though.

"I don't know what I want to do," I finally admitted. "I hate to say it, because it feels like a cop-out, but I think I just want to be a mom for a while and squeeze in some writing when I can."

"Why is that a cop-out?"

"I've made a lot of progress towards accepting that I can work and still be an attentive mom, plus we still have a lot of debt to pay back, but I think I want to be with my children more than I want to be anywhere else. I don't want to use all of my energy to save the world when the people who are most important to me right now are so young and vulnerable."

"Can you afford to stay home right now?"

"Yes... I think so. My agent says it's possible that she has another book contract for me after *Feeding the Soul* is published, and I've found that I can structure my writing so that it's flexible enough not to interfere with children. I'd like to keep running F.E.E.D. from my home and just keep sending free information out to people who need it, but I don't want to worry about getting on a plane, looking crisp and corporate, or caring about a hospital's bottom line right now. It doesn't feel like it's my calling anymore."

Kathleen and I sat together quietly. I looked out the window at the familiar scene—busy roads and perfect plots of ground. I felt Samantha kick me. Was she agreeing with me? Telling me that she wanted me around and not on a plane? She kicked again and I felt her flip.

"I've been thinking a lot about the fact that I'm going to have a daughter," I began. "Something about having a daughter, and hearing that she's going to be big like I was, has made me think about how much I want to protect her from the same comments and hurts that I went through. I want her to love herself and carry herself with pride. I want her to have all of the joy I never had. I want to launch happy children into the world—not unhealthy, unhappy people like I was."

"And you can only do that if you don't work outside the home right now?" Kathleen was trying to get to the point.

"I want to work, but I want to do it on my own terms, and I want to figure out what exactly that means without any pressure. I love to write, but it doesn't exactly make a lot of money, so I'd like to explore other fields when I'm ready. I'm almost thirty, and half of my life has now either been struggling with bulimia or recovering from it and helping others recover from it. I'm tired. I want to focus on my family. It's time to go private again and mostly just be Caroline the mom and wife. I think it's what will make me happy right now." I couldn't ignore the internal neon sign that had been flashing at me for weeks, signaling that I needed to change directions. This felt like the right way to go, and I was going to trust my intuition again and hope for the best because when I'd followed that course, my inner wisdom had never been wrong.

* * * * * * * *

IRONICALLY, I WAS looking at tall women as my water broke around midnight of July 30th, 1992. I knew something had just happened when I felt a distinctive internal "pop" while the 1992 Olympic volleyball match played on the television in front of me. Samantha was ready to make her debut.

A few weeks earlier, on a particularly hot and sweaty day, during which I'd sat in front of an air conditioner in the hopes of cooling myself off, I'd ended the day with a strange dream in which I'd gone into a store to pick her up. The clerk had reached behind the counter and opened a shoebox that said, "Miller" on the outside. "She's not cooked yet," he'd said after glancing into the box and replacing it on the shelf. Tonight, however, Samantha was finally cooked and ready to leave the shoebox known as my stomach.

Fortunately, the hospital where I'd given birth to Haywood was only a few miles from our condo, so within fifteen minutes I was entering the doors of Union Memorial Hospital, familiar with the drill that lay ahead. Eight painful hours later, my gorgeous daughter arrived, long and big as predicted, and weighing over 9-½ pounds. She was strangely quiet, but when I saw my husband's face light up, I knew that she was perfect, with no Wellbutrin deformities. An immediate father-daughter love affair was launched, with Haywood being the first to bathe our new daughter.

Samantha was fine, I heard over and over again. My daughter was healthy and well. I closed my eyes and said a prayer of thanks. I had my boy and my girl, and I was done with baby-making. Pregnancy was a risky undertaking, and I was grateful that I'd been blessed twice now. Whew.

On Kathleen's advice, I let a few weeks pass before telling the hospital chain that I wasn't interested in working with them any longer. The unit was doing well, but I was crystal-clear that my own children needed me more than anyone in any other city needed me, and also that I needed them. In addition, I wanted to be the mother I'd always wanted to have, and those efforts would occupy every bit of my strength and time.

Haywood was ambivalent about my choice. He knew that I wanted to contribute to the family's bottom line and that we could use my income to help pay down the debt, but it was possible to make it without my salary and we also wouldn't have to worry about the costs of childcare. "Do what makes you happy," he said. "You never really had a chance to enjoy being a mother when Haywood was born because of what we were going through, and it would be nice to at least experience an infant without so many distractions."

It was bittersweet to call Jill and announce my plans. She didn't try to argue with me, and agreed that if my heart wasn't in working outside the home at that time, and I wasn't up for significant travel, then it wasn't a good fit for them either.

I hung up and looked at the bassinet where Samantha lay soundly asleep. Haywood was at his pre-school and the condo was completely silent, except for my daughter's soft, steady breathing.

Something else was out there for me, but I had no idea what it was. All I knew was that my intuition was telling me that my work with the eating disorder field was over for now, and that I had had the closure I needed to my Renewal dreams by shepherding the hospital unit into being. I could move forward confidently now, and carve out whatever I wanted my destiny to be, professionally and personally. The first thirty years were now behind me, and they had been eventful, passionate and challenging years. What would the next thirty hold?

I had an inkling of just how different my life could be, but first I'd have to weather the deepest and most poignant challenges I'd ever faced in defining myself as an independent, recovering woman. It would be in a place I knew only too well. Ground Zero was calling.

## CHAPTER FOURTEEN
## THE LEANING TOWER OF PISA

When my first child, Haywood, was born, everything in our lives went haywire immediately. In quick succession, my husband and I lost our home, our money, and a major professional dream. The only thing that saved us on many days was that we had a son whom we adored, and whose personality lit up dark days and gave us a reason to keep pushing forward, regardless of the bad news that kept rolling in.

After giving birth, I'd also had to deal with the unexpected side effects of losing too much weight and needing to learn how to gain it back, plus confronting some of the underlying issues around the way I'd been raised and the impact some of those issues had continued to have on me as an adult and a mother. Going on antidepressants and getting back into therapy had been a major step for me in broadening my recovery experience, as had being part of a challenging introspective group therapy process where I'd learned more about the dynamics of healthy relationships. None of this had been easy, particularly with almost no money in the bank, and stranded in a town where we barely knew anyone, but I'd found the resources I needed, had done the work, and we had all survived and somehow thrived.

Samantha's birth seemed to have the opposite effect on our lives: everything that had gone wrong for us three years earlier now went incredibly well. Instead of being bankrupt and homeless, we were making money. Haywood's career was taking off. I had just published my second book, *Feeding the Soul*, and was running F.E.E.D. on a volunteer basis in my spare time. Most positively, instead of greeting every day with a certain amount of dread, we regularly awoke in our Baltimore condo excited to face the possibilities of each day.

Our life now had a soothing and predictable rhythm. Haywood routinely departed by 7 a.m. for his job in Washington, D.C., and returned by 7 p.m., while I occupied myself with cleaning, cooking and caring for the children, squeezing in a few minutes here and there to write ideas for my next book. Young Haywood was in a partial-day preschool in the Baltimore suburbs that gave him room to run and lots of playground activity, and I was fortunate to find a young high school graduate who helped me with Samantha for a few hours a day when I needed to go out or just enjoy a few quiet hours. The balance felt right: I was satisfied as a writer, mother and wife. Life was good again.

Just as the domino effect of bad news in 1989 had created a downward spiral of wellbeing, the domino effect of good news now spiraled us upwards, with seemingly endless positive outcomes. Haywood's company was named the top performer in the American Stock Exchange in 1992 and the value of our stock skyrocketed. His mother inherited money from her parents, which she generously divided and passed along to my husband and his younger sister. After watching us career from apartment to condo to farmette to mansion to rental house and back to condo again in less than ten years, we now had the resources to try to find a more permanent place to live. The condo, which consisted of two bedrooms, one living room, and a galley kitchen, simply wasn't going to meet our needs for much longer.

Between Haywood's stock and this unexpected inheritance windfall, we paid off all of the Renewal debt in one fell swoop, eliminated our lingering college and graduate school debts, and still had enough to consider moving to a new home. What had once been unthinkable was now possible. A miracle had occurred; we felt as blessed as if we'd just found an oasis after thirstily wandering in the desert.

✳ ✳ ✳ ✳ ✳ ✳ ✳ ✳

HAYWOOD'S COMPANY HAD no intention of relocating, and my writing was portable, so we made the decision to look for homes in the Washington, D.C., area.

A real estate agent met us every weekend to show us homes within our price range all over the suburbs of Washington, D.C., primarily focused in Bethesda and Chevy Chase. On several occasions we fell in love with small three-bedroom starter homes and put in bids. Every time, however, we were outmaneuvered. Over and over we went through the bidding ritual on desirable houses, only to get a call from our disappointed agent telling us that we were, once again, on the losing end in a red-hot real estate market.

Then one night, in a blinding snowstorm, while Haywood was driving home from work, our agent reached him in his car about a new prospect that seemed to be different from everything else we'd looked at.

"Turn around and come back immediately," she ordered him. "A house went on the market tonight in the neighborhood where Caroline grew up. The owners were quite elderly, and they died without heirs, so the house is being priced by the executor for a quick sale. It's definitely going to go overnight, so get back here and let's make a bid."

Obediently, Haywood turned around and met the agent in the snow. He took a quick tour of the property and agreed to make a bid that was slightly above our price range because the house was not only perfect for us, it was a great deal. Haywood called me to say that he'd had to act quickly, but that he was sure I'd love the house if we actually got it. I agreed. It sounded ideal, and there was no way we'd lose it this time if we were bidding in the middle of the night, just hours after the house had gone on the market and before anyone else had had a chance to see it.

The following day we got a call, but not the call we had expected. Two bids had come in simultaneously: ours and the bid by a couple that had a slightly bigger down payment as part of their offer, and who had their own sharp-eyed real estate agent bidding on their behalf. We lost again.

113

I soothed myself by looking for the silver lining in these repeated losses, and particularly this last one. Was the house we'd just lost too close to my childhood homes, and we simply weren't meant to be back in that same environment? The house we had bid on was one block away from where I'd spent the first nine years of my life and two blocks away from the home where I'd spent the rest of my adolescence, including all of the years I'd battled bulimia. The park down the street was where I'd whiled away many hours swinging and playing in the trees, as well as where my grandmother had taught me how to ride my bike. The street was dotted with some of my parents' friends, and the schools I'd attended were within a few miles of the house.

Although I no longer attended group therapy, I still met with Kathleen once a week to continue our individual work. Her analysis was that I was doing very well on all fronts, and that our work was coming to a natural conclusion. She was also pleased that adding Wellbutrin back to my life after weaning Samantha appeared to be a good decision, because it seemed to optimize my brain chemistry. I no longer questioned the use of medication because this particular one had made a noticeable difference in my mood. I also believed that it had enhanced my long-term recovery from my eating disorder because my ability to sustain well-being made me less vulnerable to relapse or addiction switching.

Kathleen had also guided me through my early unease about being a working mother. She'd watched me go from writing for a few hours while Haywood went to family daycare, to tentatively reclaiming a professional identity by working with the hospital chain. Despite how far I'd come in that area, though, it was never easy. Every working mother I knew had some conflicting feelings around pursuing her own dreams, particularly when the children were small. We were damned if we worked and damned if we didn't. If we worked out of necessity, there was often guilt about not being with our kids and anger that the choice hadn't even been ours. Working for pleasure and leaving childcare primarily to sitters left us open to judgment and occasional doubts about being selfish. Writing offered me the best compromise to this dilemma that I could think of: I didn't have to travel, I didn't have to leave my home to be productive, and I was keeping my brain occupied while making money during a few selected hours of the day.

Because Kathleen knew me as well as I knew myself, and could often see pitfalls before I did, I knew she'd have a good take on our latest losing real estate bid.

"We almost got a house that is very close to where my parents live," I told her a few days later during our session. "Although I know it's necessary to be closer to where Haywood works, I wonder if we lost the house because I'm not supposed to re-experience some of the memories I have from my childhood, or see my parents as regularly as I would if they were right around the block. You know how hard it's been for me to even visit my grandmother in my childhood home."

"That could be," Kathleen responded carefully, "but you may still have more digging to do around your relationship with them, even though you're holding your own now. Once you move back anywhere near where you grew up, some issues you're not aware of could emerge, particularly as your children hit the ages that remind you of painful times in your own life. Things have a way of coming up when it's time for them to come up; remember the Leaning Tower of Pisa analogy where you see the same scene from different vantage points the higher you climb? You may have to revisit therapy at those times."

"Hmmm...." I didn't like that thought. As much as I appreciated the good things that emerged from working with Kathleen and my previous therapist, I wanted to be done with therapy. It was hard, expensive, and time-consuming. How much more could there be to work through? I'd spent hours and hours excavating my memories with Kathleen, sorting through the pain and rearranging my brain so that I could have healthier reactions whenever I was triggered by anything or anyone. There had to be a finish line.

In an unexpected development, the couple that had unexpectedly snatched the house away from us backed out within a week. They were relocating from the Midwest, and when they actually saw the house that the real estate agent had bid on for them, they were horrified by how little their money bought in the Washington area, compared to where they currently lived. They wanted to keep looking. The house went back on the market and we had another shot.

We pounced. Because of my background and knowledge of the area, I knew that the house was actually underpriced relative to the Washington market, so we rebid on the house and went over the asking price, determined not to lose this time. We won, despite the fact that the bidding pool was now even larger.

My parents and grandmother excitedly met us at the house we were going to move into in the spring of 1993. Their happiness, and excitement about being closer to our children, seemed genuine. Had I changed so much that my parents wouldn't trigger me? Had they changed, too? I couldn't tell and didn't have those answers, but I decided to take peace and proximity to my grandmother over any concerns about being in my childhood neighborhood and near my family. We made plans to move around Easter 1993 with our almost-four-year-old son and young daughter. I was going to be back home, and this time was going to be different. Or at least that's what I told myself.

# CHAPTER FIFTEEN
## THE RIGHT PATH?

Westmoreland Hills is undeniably beautiful, and the day we moved in, a perfect day by Washington, D.C., standards, made the neighborhood look even more serene. Azalea bushes were beginning to burst open with the vibrant hues of pink, orange and white dotting most front yards, including ours. Weeping cherry and magnolia trees were budding up and down the street. Our house was situated on top of a hill, with the vista in each direction affording us a priceless view. The house had a loving vibration that everyone felt when they walked in the door; the prior owners had been devoted to each other, and our neighbors all told us stories of their kindness. The house had been their child, and they had lavished their attention on every detail. I felt like this couple had somehow wanted us to be the second owners of this special house, and that our move was predestined. It had to be good, I told myself. My neon internal sign flashed "Right way!"

Instead of leaving Baltimore without a proper set of goodbyes, this time we were determined to preserve our friendships by staying in close touch. All of my self-help group friends had my new phone number and an open invitation to visit any time. Kathleen and I agreed that the difficulties of getting to her office from Washington in the middle of the day, as well as our shared feeling that I was doing well, had brought us to appropriate closure. There were no current crises in my life and I was content. I was proud of myself; I was a stronger, better version of the woman who had written *My Name is Caroline.*

I'd gone from once thinking that I'd have my eating disorder hovering around me for the rest of my life, waiting to grab me because of my addictive nature, to feeling completely healed. I was confident and had no fears of relapse. Was I completely cured? I didn't know, but it sure felt like it. What had once seemed impossible was now reality, and I was proud to return to my hometown, and even my old neighborhood, as a completely healed and transformed adult woman.

* * * * * * * *

OUR FIRST YEAR back in Bethesda passed in a flurry of activities—finding new doctors and dentists, reconnecting with childhood friends, getting involved in local activities with the children. Watching my children's personalities unfold was one of my greatest delights, which I often noted in my journals. I had also started a tradition when Haywood was born of writing each child a letter on their "birth day," as well as on each subsequent birthday. In these handwritten, multi-page letters I poured out my love for Haywood and Samantha, what we hoped their lives would hold, and what they were doing and experiencing—their first words, steps or friendships.

Haywood was quick in every way. He'd always been hard to keep up with from an energy perspective, which I'd just assumed was part of raising a red-blooded, athletic boy. In fact, whenever we were in public, his favorite game was to run away as fast as he could. We'd learned to tie a balloon to his wrist so that if he escaped while we were distracted with Samantha, one of us could easily spot him and recapture him. Strollers had never worked with our son; he wouldn't sit down long enough to be walked anywhere peacefully, and since he'd outgrown the Jolly Jumper, we knew that we had to be especially vigilant when we were in public. We'd had a few close calls, though. The only time I'd ever spanked Haywood was when he decided to run full-speed towards an intersection with moving traffic, simply because he wanted to see how fast he could go, and no one was going to stop him.

In addition to moving quickly, Haywood thought quickly. From the time he was two, he would take any puzzle and put it together with lightning speed, contentedly sucking on two fingers to celebrate the completion of his efforts. Lincoln Log houses were assembled in the blink of an eye. By the age of four, despite the fact that he wasn't yet reading, he had memorized the order and all of the names of United States presidents, which he would recite to any adult who cared to listen.

Samantha was a very different child. She was more cautious, taking in everything with her eyes before risking getting involved. Where Haywood flung himself headlong into life, Samantha held back and waited to understand the lay of the land before making a move. She was also a happy child, but in a quieter way. One thing that brought her tremendous joy manifested early in the form of creating order in her environment. For example, one day I found her straightening all of the tassels on the Oriental rug on the landing outside her room, refusing to descend the stairs until they were all perfectly separated and straight.

Both children had their quirks and strengths, but their energies were complementary and our house was harmonious in almost every respect. My parents kept a respectful distance, which led me to believe that they had overcome whatever problems they'd once had with me, and that I'd been foolish to think that my childhood issues with them would rear their head in my thirties. Not only was I in recovery from my eating disorder, but I was also in recovery from my childhood demons. This satisfying stage of development, I decided, was the reward for all of my years of deep, internal work.

* * * * * * * *

BEFORE WE KNEW IT, Haywood and I were grappling with the issue of where to send our children to school. I had attended a string of private schools, from preschool through high school, while my husband had mostly attended public schools Virginia, New York, New Jersey, and Maryland. We had both wound up in the same place, my husband had once noted, so he didn't support the notion that expensive private schools were the only way to go if

119

getting a good education was a priority. He'd reached Harvard without his parents spending much money on schools, while I'd never been in a tax-supported classroom in my life. Was I more intelligent, better-educated and world-savvy than he was because of the different emphasis in my family on schooling?

Haywood certainly didn't think so. Once he had cynically observed, "You read *Bleak House* in eighth grade and I read it in my twenties—is that really worth spending $200,000 after-tax dollars on private schools for each child now that we've just gotten out of debt?" He had a way of isolating the key factor of any argument we were having. His simplified comparison of my education versus his wasn't exactly accurate, but he had made his point and made me laugh at the same time.

Technically, I agreed with Haywood about the insanity of private school costs. If Montgomery County, one of the wealthiest counties in the country, containing some of the most well-educated people in America, didn't have good public schools, who did? My class composition at Harvard argued in favor of looking at public schools, too, because over 60% of my classmates had come from public schools.

Now we were facing a decision: should we send our son Haywood to our local elementary school or throw in our lot with the private school treadmill, which, I knew, didn't easily let you off once you'd gotten aboard. If a child's friendships and learning coalesced around a certain school, it was jarring to switch midstream, which is why so many of the private schools in town had pre-schools that hooked into specific grade schools, some of which went from kindergarten through high school. Getting over the admissions hurdle and winning the brass ring for a ride through high school was dearly coveted by many families.

I still wondered if I should at least go through the private school applications process for Haywood. Was it selfish to deny him any chance of having the same excellent education I'd had without even considering it? Would he be behind the curve if we didn't offer him the same opportunities I'd had? For all of my parents' flaws, they had worked to ensure that their three children all had first-class educations. This wasn't a decision I wanted to make lightly.

Haywood and I came to a standoff on the public vs. private issue as our son approached kindergarten age and we had to make a choice. Our compromise was that I agreed to look at the local public school with an open mind. My husband agreed to have Haywood apply to the same school I'd attended, but with the caveat that we would only send him there if he got in and it was unquestionably the best environment for his energy level and intellect.

The Norwood School, which I had attended, had been in the dusty rented rooms of a church when I was a student; now it looked like a country club in verdant horse country. As we toured the impressive, lush grounds dotted with lacrosse nets and well-watered playing fields, I wondered how we'd ever made do on the blacktop of yore. The interior of the school was just as jaw-dropping; no expense had been spared in the art rooms, music auditorium, theater, language labs and carpeted classrooms. A child wanted for nothing here.

The price tag was over-the-top too. Kindergarten started at $15,000 and the cost would continue to climb, the admissions director informed us, plus we were expected to donate to the Annual Giving fund. Haywood looked shocked as we took in the surroundings, occasionally whispering that Harvard hadn't held a candle to some of the amenities we saw.

On the way home we talked about our reactions.

"I'm not convinced it's the right place after seeing how ridiculously perfect it is, plus we just can't afford it C," he said decisively. "If we send Haywood there, it is the equivalent of buying one car every year for thirteen years."

I couldn't disagree. I kept thinking back to my own years at Norwood, though. I had been so alive there. I had literally devoured books, been absorbed by the teaching, and made some of my best friends there, including Anne. I'd always had a teacher ready to explain something to me, and had received my first intellectual awakenings there. Instead of feeling unloved or unwanted, I'd always felt special at school, and had become hooked on the joy of education. I was also regularly told I was smart, and no one ever told me to stop asking questions.

"I still want Haywood to apply," I said, staring glumly out the window. "How can you deny that he'd blossom physically and educationally there? He'd have recess twice a day, small classes that could accommodate his energy level, and stimulation from every direction. I can't even imagine how much he'd get here, even though it definitely comes across as way over the top. I don't disagree with you about that."

We rode in silence the rest of the way home. As we entered our neighborhood, Haywood offered an olive branch.

"Okay, we'll apply if you will regret not doing it," Haywood conceded. "And I know you loved it there. But I still think it's a hell of a lot of money. Don't forget that we have to earn twice as much as what it costs because this is all after-tax money, and then you can double that figure, too, because we can't do something for Haywood that we're not prepared to do for Samantha."

He was right. But we didn't have to cross that bridge yet, so we just decided to get Haywood tested and see if admission was even in the cards.

# CHAPTER SIXTEEN
## MISS DIAGNOSIS

The envelope arrived in the spring. After months of waiting, here was the letter from Norwood containing news of our son's fate. Weren't thin letters a sign of rejection? Or was that only for college? I was nervous as I ripped into the letter.

"Congratulations! We are delighted to offer Haywood a spot in the incoming kindergarten class," the letter opened. It went on to spell out how long we had to accept or reject the offer, along with a hefty deposit we'd have to send in if we agreed to join them.

The last paragraph was a bit unusual, though. "As delightful as your son is, we believe he needs to be evaluated for hyperactivity, and we'd like you to call the physician we refer to in situations like this. If he believes that Haywood has attention-deficit hyperactivity disorder, as we suspect, we must stipulate that he only attend the school on medication."

Huh? There was a condition to this acceptance letter? And it involved possibly putting my child on medication if we wanted to accept the offer?

I had several strong reactions. First off, I'd never seen or heard of anything like this type of acceptance for an elementary school, although I'd certainly seen it during my senior year in high school. I knew several people who had been accepted to specific Ivy League schools that boasted buildings or endowments from the student's family, but the child in question simply didn't fit the bill for the school's criteria. "You may come to the college in the fall, but we don't think it's in your best interests to do so," I remembered one letter announcing to a boy in my social circle.

After my initial reaction of shock to Norwood's letter, I became angry. What were these people talking about? My son was plenty bright, and all boys were as active as Haywood was. Medication to level the playing field so that I could grab onto happiness was one thing, but medication to change a young child's energy level? That would destroy the lovable essence of who he was. As tired as I often was at the end of the day, I loved the fact that Haywood lit up our house with verve and enthusiasm. There was never a dull moment when he was around.

My husband was equally annoyed. "How do you like the part about the fact that they pick the doctor *for* you?" he scoffed as he perused the letter. "Just beautiful. We'll be sent to some doctor where the outcome is already fixed. This is offensive," he said, tossing the letter aside. "You don't accept a kid and put conditions on it—you take them or you don't take them. It's that simple."

Since I was the one with a history with the school and a relationship with the director, I offered to call Jill for clarification. Perhaps there was a misunderstanding. Maybe they meant something else, although I couldn't imagine another way to interpret being told that your child needed a medical evaluation to be considered worthy.

I got Jill on the first try. "Congratulations on Haywood's admission!" she said. "What can I help you with today?"

"Well," I started, not wanting to offend her or lose Haywood's spot at this school. "We were a little surprised by the wording in the letter about the doctor and the possibility of putting Haywood on medication."

"Oh, of course," she said quickly. "You need Dr. Hammerman's number, don't you? I think we forgot to put it in the letter. Let me get it for you." With that, I was put on hold until she reappeared with a bright voice and the contact information.

"Thank you," I stammered. "But we were actually wondering why you only give one name, and why you felt this was necessary at all."

Jill then went into a long explanation about how this particular doctor had written the most widely-accepted textbooks on the various attention deficit disorders, primarily Attention Deficit Hyperactivity Disorder (ADHD) which the school's testers suspected Haywood had, and Attention Deficit Disorder (ADD), which was a completely different diagnosis. Jill said that we were fortunate to have one of the foremost experts in the world in our area, which was why the school referred to him so often in a case like this. After hearing what she had to say, I didn't disagree. He sounded like a scholar and a thorough doctor.

"But what exactly did Haywood do during the testing that brought this all about?" I pressed. "Aren't all boys as active as he is? Is he really so different? Or do you have a lot of kids on medication at the school?"

"Caroline," Jill said with a laugh. "It was apparent to the testers that your son is very bright, but they had to cut short almost every evaluation because he wouldn't stay put long enough to finish any of them. Have you ever noticed that he doesn't sit still for very long?"

Had I ever noticed that my child didn't sit still? Was she kidding? I felt like saying something inappropriate, so I chose my next words carefully.

"Sure, I've noticed, but so what? This school has such a low student-teacher ratio that you are ideal for a situation like this where a child can always be kept busy and get enough attention, right? One of the reasons why we wanted to apply to the school was precisely because of his energy level, and because the tuition ought to cover that type of one-on-one instruction. Going to the public schools means bigger classes and less time with organized sports and activities. Isn't this exactly the kind of thing you are designed to handle better than anyone else without putting a kid on pills?"

I suddenly felt like I was pleading with the school, hoping that they would see Haywood as a normal child, at least by their standards. This acceptance letter actually felt like a rejection to me, and I was frantically trying to turn it around.

There was a long pause. "Caroline, our teachers are first-class, but Haywood is one of the most hyperactive children we've ever evaluated. Even in a small class, he'd be too much for a teacher to handle."

I was chastened into silence and felt old fears of unworthiness come upon me, but not because of anything I'd done. My son was in the "yes but" category because of his energy level, and the same school where I'd thrived, and where I'd also had a high energy level, only wanted *my* kid with conditions. I felt like this was suddenly a secret club and we didn't know the right handshake to get in the door.

Maybe Haywood *was* more hyperactive than other kids, but how much? I didn't want him to get a reputation for being difficult, however I needed some basis for comparison. I said we'd meet with the doctor they recommended to get a diagnosis and we'd get back to them.

Less than a week later, Haywood and I met with Dr. Hammerman, who did indeed have an impressive list of credentials, articles, books, and appointments that designated him as one of the premier experts in the areas of attention disorders. He confessed that some of his interest in the topic stemmed from having been diagnosed with ADHD himself.

"Does that make you even more likely to diagnose a child with this disorder?" my husband asked. He was still a little angry that we'd been given only one option to go to for a diagnosis that the school would accept, and he was convinced that it was because the doctor was pill-happy and the school wanted sedated kids.

Dr. Hammerman surprised us with his answer. "Actually, I disappoint more parents than you can imagine by NOT giving them an ADHD or ADD diagnosis. A lot of them are hoping that their child will get medication that will make them quiet and easy to manage, in addition to the fact that the schools give you testing accommodations if you have this diagnosis. Sometimes it's all about giving their kid an edge in a competitive town, and I won't go along with it. If you don't have it, you don't have it, and I'm not about to make it up so that some kid can get untimed testing for SATs in high school."

THAT surprised us. Untimed testing for SATs? What a thought! I'd never heard of such a thing, and Dr. Hammerman's response wasn't what we had expected. A week later, after his evaluation with our son, we had our results.

"Mr. and Mrs. Miller," Dr. Hammerman said, opening the folder containing notes about our child, "Haywood is off the charts, and my opinion is that he has one of the most pronounced cases of ADHD that I've ever seen. It's not even a close call." He gave us a few more details about the testing, and how he'd come to his conclusion, and then he recommended that we start a medication trial with Ritalin to see how he reacted. "Stimulant medication is in and out of your bloodstream in four hours, and it will work or it won't. You'll know if it is effective immediately."

No kidding? No half-life to the medication, and no building it up in your bloodstream to see if it worked? The instant gratification was definitely appealing when I compared it to my extended Prozac episode. Dr. Hammerman went on to say that stimulant medication had been used safely and effectively for decades, and that the only side-effect we might see would be a reduced appetite. He also noted that children like Haywood who were appropriately diagnosed and given the right medication at a young age had been found to be less likely to abuse illegal drugs and alcohol as they got older.

"Where does a condition like this come from?" I asked. I was truly a babe in the woods on this topic; I hadn't had time to read any books about ADHD because everything had moved so quickly. I'd figured that I would learn more if Haywood actually had the diagnosis.

"It's genetic," Dr. Hammerman said simply. "It must be in one or both of your families. Do you have relatives who are like Haywood, and who are very hyperactive?"

"My dad is like that," my husband answered. "He probably hasn't read a single book in his whole life, but he's really smart. He was at the top of his class at the Naval Academy in math. Does ADHD mean you aren't smart?"

"No, quite the contrary," Dr. Hammerman reassured us. "These kids with ADHD often become the class presidents, football quarterbacks and successful entrepreneurs, on top of being very intelligent. If you diagnose and treat the condition early, you can channel the energy into all kinds of productive areas. The medication just makes it easier for you to sit and focus on things that *don't* necessarily interest you, but that you still have to do."

"So you're not saying that our son is stupid," I said, "just that he has a battery that he has to tame, particularly so that he can sit through some of the things in school that don't necessarily grab his interest."

"Exactly. And as he gets older, you'll find that it makes socializing with peers easier. Not many people can keep up with someone with ADHD because they can overwhelm others with their intensity and energy. You don't want your child to experience that type of rejection if you can avoid it with the proper medication."

As Dr. Hammerman outlined the life of a child with ADHD, I had the eerie feeling that he was talking about me, and not just my son. His words sounded just like how I'd always been described by friends, family and teachers. Was it possible that I had this condition, too?

"This actually sounds a lot like me," I hesitantly offered. "Is it possible that I have ADHD, too, and that maybe Haywood got it from me?" After all, my son took after my blond side of the family, and I'd been told that we had the same mannerisms, and even that we walked like each other. Had he inherited my brain, too?

"Of course it's possible. In fact, I wouldn't be surprised if you have ADHD, but you never knew it. Sometimes it's the primary diagnosis in a child, but if it's not identified and treated, other behaviors may emerge, such as depression, cutting and eating disorders. Didn't you say that you had bulimia at one time?"

Did I have yet another condition that might require medication? And was he saying that my eating disorder might be a secondary condition that could have arisen because the ADHD had never been recognized and treated? My brain spun as I thought about these possibilities. I asked Dr. Hammerman if I could have an appointment for myself as soon as possible to test me for ADHD, and then we left. I felt like I'd just been hit by a truck.

I made a beeline for the phone when I got home to call my parents and ask them some questions. I got my dad on the first ring.

I explained the reason for my call and mentioned that the doctor thought that I might have ADHD, too, which might have been apparent when I was a child.

"Did anyone ever tell you and Mom that I had an attention issue when I was younger, or that I might be hyperactive?"

"Yes," he said immediately. "The doctor gave us some pills when you were young, and we used them for about a week, but we didn't think they worked. We threw them out and decided not to worry about it. We were also concerned about the stigma of having a daughter on medication, and how it would be perceived by people if they found out."

"So I was diagnosed with hyperactivity when I was younger, and no one ever told me? Or did much of anything about it?" I asked in wonderment.

I was also digesting the fact that they'd been worried about the stigma of having a daughter on medication. Had they been concerned about it because of their own reputations, or because of mine? I had so many questions I wanted to ask, but knew that I'd probably get nowhere if I was perceived as blaming them, particularly if I said there was a connection between undiagnosed ADHD and developing an eating disorder. They had taken the resolute position for years that they'd had zero role in the development of my eating disorder. They would never budge from that place, nor did I expect them to.

"Yes, but you did just fine, didn't you?" my dad replied mildly. "You swam fast, excelled in school, and went to Harvard. How bad an outcome is that?"

Actually, it was one that I wished I had known about a long time ago. I spent every waking minute the following week reading through the books and literature about ADHD. I fit *every* criteria for the disorder, just like my son, and now that I was 32, I was realizing that my impatience, impulsiveness, and inability to do something as simple as sit through a movie might actually be due to my brain chemistry, much like my inability to keep my happiness levels up at times.

As I read through the descriptions of how the brains of people with ADHD differ from others, the word "dopamine" stood out to me. I had been unable to tolerate Prozac, leading me to try Wellbutrin, which blocked the reuptake of dopamine from receptor cells. Now I was learning that ADHD was also linked with dopamine deficiencies. It all fell into place. When it came to processing dopamine, my body was a dud.

I was particularly interested in what the literature said about frequent co-existence of bulimia with ADHD. If stimulant medication worked for ADHD, it would help to explain why I had started drinking gallons and gallons of coffee at a young age. Instead of making me jittery and revving me up, coffee had the opposite effect of calming me down. Another thing that had always had a sedative effect on me was binging and purging, which I'd read somewhere had the impact of flooding the brain with dopamine.

Had I been unwittingly trying to fix my brain chemistry myself and create extra dopamine wherever I could find it, getting stuck in behaviors that partly alleviated my condition, but ultimately brought more harm than good? Could all of this have been eliminated if my parents had simply persevered in keeping me on medication when a doctor told them I was hyperactive, regardless of what anyone else thought of them?

Now, twenty-seven years after that first diagnosis of hyperactivity, and just days after Dr. Hammerman had seconded it, I was reflecting back on my life, wondering if so many of the difficulties I'd faced could have been avoided by my parents paying closer attention to a doctor when I was a child, and making sure that I had had medication, if necessary, for a condition that had the tendency to sprout side-effects if left untreated. It was obvious that my needs had gone unaddressed. The price I'd paid for this omission was just starting to come into focus, and it was staggering.

\* \* \* \* \* \* \* \*

MY SON AND I started Ritalin on the same day. Our mornings usually began before 6 a.m., which wasn't unusual, because that's when five-year-old

Haywood usually bounded out of bed, chattering and looking for things to do. Dr. Hammerman had told us that many parents with ADHD children installed televisions in their bedrooms to keep their children occupied until more normal hours, but I was usually up by then myself. Haywood and I had also agreed that television in our children's bedrooms would never happen because there wouldn't be an incentive for them to turn it off. Dr. Hammerman had also suggested getting a huge clock with digital times so that we could teach Haywood to stay put until the number said 7. No dice.

One of Haywood's favorite early morning activities was to practice his batting swing in the backyard, the moment the sun came up. He was heading out the door when I intercepted him and told him that we were starting an experiment with some tiny pills that might make him feel a little bit different. Dr. Hammerman had given us the lingo to use with a child around beginning medication. He said to be matter-of-fact and to avoid making it a big deal. He advised that the child be coached to treat Ritalin like a Cheerio, and to place it on the back of the tongue for ease in swallowing. I did all of those things and Haywood immediately swallowed the pill.

I didn't know exactly what to expect, so I just sat down and observed him from the kitchen window. Haywood did his normal baseball routine for about ten minutes, running around imaginary bases after swinging at invisible baseballs. Just as I was wondering if I'd see any impact, he did the unthinkable: he put the bat down and walked inside the house. I'd never seen him stop doing anything physical before getting tired, so this was a new development. I was riveted.

He came in the door and went right up to his room. I followed and hovered at his door, making small talk, trying to figure out what was happening. Then Haywood took a huge stack of baseball cards and began to sort them methodically, putting them in piles of teams. I watched, fascinated. He finished that job and moved onto another organizational project that involved counting. Although he was quieter and more focused than normal, my son didn't appear to be a zombie, much to my relief. He giggled and laughed when it was appropriate. When it was time to go to the pre-school, which was right up the street, he gathered his belongings and went obediently, without any last-minute forgetfulness.

As I walked Haywood to school and came back home, I thought about what I had just witnessed. There had, indeed, been an immediate impact when I'd given Haywood the Ritalin. It was almost as if a switch had been flipped, ordering him to cease excessive physical activity and to focus on something. That something had been baseball cards, but in a school setting, it would obviously be a class. I could see why teachers would want kids to be on this medication.

Now it was my turn to try the drug. I swallowed it and sat down in the kitchen. I felt like someone from the 1960s who had taken LSD and wanted to be a participant in their own trip. Within just a few minutes, I felt something akin to a blip in my brain, almost like a stream of bubbles that burst from a hidden spring. As I began to go about my morning, including taking care of Samantha and doing some writing, the only analogy I could think of was that I'd gone from 90 miles per hour to a more reasonable 65. Much as I'd felt the first time I tried Wellbutrin, this reaction to a drug felt very right. Something in my brain suddenly felt like the kinks had been worked out. I was amazed.

By the time Haywood came home that afternoon, the medication had worn off, for both of us. He was his usual active self, wanting to go in ten directions at once, which was something I often wanted to do myself, and he didn't seem to have had any negative impact from spending a few hours on medication. It gradually dawned on me that I may have written off Haywood's energy level as "normal" all these years simply because it matched mine, and that I hadn't been able to identify his hyperactivity for what it really was because I had never identified it in myself. I'd enjoyed at least four hours of feeling completely organized and focused and clear-headed in a new and different way, and it had been an eye-opener. If his morning had been anything like mine, it had been a blessing.

Before we made any long-term decision about staying on the medication, though, I wanted to collect more data about how Haywood had

132

behaved at school. I called his teachers and told them I'd given him a trial dose of Ritalin that morning, and asked if they'd noticed anything different about him.

"I'm so glad you asked," Margaret said. Margaret was the founder and long-time teacher at the small Montessori pre-school and had educated hundreds of children over many years. She knew her stuff, and I was sure she'd be right on the money with any of her reactions. "It certainly explains what we observed." I braced myself. Was this going to be positive?

"Haywood sat down and *read* a book for the first time this morning," she said. "He obviously knew specific words before today, but we'd never seen him sit down and immerse himself in a book and read it from start to finish himself."

I had the image of a child who'd had discrete concepts swirling through his head for a long time, but who had never had the ability to quiet himself and put them all together. Dr. Hammerman had told us that the impact of the Ritalin would be immediate, and it had been. I was a convert. If my son could pull together ideas and apply them with focus within hours of a small dose of Ritalin, and have the world of reading suddenly available to him, I could only imagine the other benefits that awaited him in his future.

I called Dr. Hammerman and told him about our reactions to the medication, and said that the trial was already over in my mind because my son and I had instantly seen the benefits. Delighted but not surprised, he told me that he'd write us both prescriptions for the next month, but that we'd need to transfer our future care for medication to our regular doctors. He also told me something I'd already suspected—that the Wellbutrin and Ritalin would probably work in harmony and even amplify each other's effects. He said that the Wellbutrin would assist me further with focus, and that the Ritalin would probably enhance my well-being because they both acted on the dopamine pathways.

I felt, deep in my gut, that I now had the level chemical playing field that had always eluded me, and that I had just given birth to a new way of life. While I'd been successful in many arenas, I'd always felt like something was missing, and that I'd had to work harder than other people to do something as simple as focus, be happy, or develop resilience. Perhaps I'd simply needed to have my brain chemistry tweaked to handle life more effectively. I vowed that although I had missed out on this for my first 32 years, I was going to enjoy whatever lay in front of me with this brain cocktail that appeared to be a winner.

Maybe it was the clarity brought about by the Ritalin, or maybe it was just a negative reaction to Norwood's acceptance letter, but my husband and I decided that the school was not the right place for our child and we would not be sending Haywood there for kindergarten. We didn't doubt that it offered a great education, and nothing would ever extinguish my wonderful memories of being a student there, but something about pigeonholing our child from the get-go and telling us that they'd only take him as a medicated student had caused us to think twice. Now that I knew I'd had ADHD as a student there, I wondered why the school had the ability to handle me, but not my son. Did they not want their teachers to work too hard, or be creative in the ways they dealt with active students? Did they just want the easy way out?

Maybe a high-energy, inquisitive child, like I'd been, could add some innovative pizzazz to a classroom instead of disrupting it. Maybe there was nothing wrong with us, but something was wrong with them. It was a powerful insight, and one that represented a significant break with the "right school" mentality I'd been raised with. Public school was good enough for the majority of the world, and it was going to be good enough for my children. They didn't have to do four hours of homework every night or read Charles Dickens earlier than their peers; they would be just fine at the rest of the world's pace. "Right Way!" flashed frantically.

I felt a sense of peace descend on the house as I made this decision without worrying about how it would be perceived by anyone else. Instead of repeating my own educational path, I was going to break new ground for myself and my children and do something completely different from how I'd been raised. Perhaps it wouldn't work out perfectly, but most things never did, anyway, and I was game to see how it would all play out.

Then, just as so many other peaceful times in my life had played out, everything abruptly turned upside-down, marking the onset of the most extraordinarily difficult, but ultimately healing, chapters in my recovery. Although I'd thought that I'd reached the pinnacle of inner development and joy when I moved back into my old neighborhood, little did I know that it had just been the appetizer to the main meal.

## CHAPTER SEVENTEEN
## CAN CHAOS LEAD TO ORDER?

I stared at the white plastic stick in disbelief. Here I was again, in a bathroom, alone, staring at a piece of plastic that had just changed my life in the space of a heartbeat.

I wasn't happy or unhappy, I noted dully, sitting on the edge of a toilet and looking out the window. Stunned was more like it.

When Haywood and I had moved into this brick, center hall Colonial in Westmoreland Hills a year earlier—the house of our dreams—we'd felt like we'd found the perfect place to raise our completed, nuclear family. We had our boy and our girl and we were done making babies. We were out of debt, contented, and life was good.

Now, against all odds, and the enthusiastic use of birth control, I was clearly pregnant again. Nausea? Check. Exhaustion? Check. Weird metal taste in my mouth? Check. This plastic stick with a pretty pink line was the *coup de grace.* "Here we go again," I wearily thought.

I sighed. Why did my life have this unmistakable pattern of calm followed by upheaval, topped off by a frantic paddling back to shore to save myself and make sense of it all? Someone had once told me that order only emerged from chaos, but I truly didn't want any more chaos at the moment because I was satisfied with the current order.

This particular kind of health risk had also been one that I'd had no intention of ever taking again, which was why I was so careful. Every pregnancy was a roll of the dice, in my opinion, and we'd been extremely fortunate. I loved the fact that I had two totally different children, one of each, healthy, and nicely spaced. So much for intelligent planning!

I got to my feet. It was time to tell Haywood, once again by telephone, that he was going to be a father. There was no way I could keep the news from him, or even conceal this explosive knowledge if he checked in during the day. I was terrible at hiding information anyway, so I always figured that I should get announcements like this over with as quickly as possible.

"Haywood—I have something interesting to tell you." There wasn't a clever way to tell my husband he had helped to start the parenthood train again, so I stuck with the basics.

"Okay," he said, knowing from experience that lives can change with a single phone call. "What?"

"I'm pregnant."

The silence at the other end of the phone said it all. I stumbled on.

"We're going to have another baby. Next February, I think."

It was early July now, and I was probably five weeks along. As I thought back to when I might have conceived, I remembered what my son had said to me when he turned five in early May.

"What do you want for your birthday, honey?"

Although I had a pretty good idea about what Haywood liked, it was still fun to have conversations like this to see if I learned something new about a toy craze I hadn't heard about yet. Also, in the month that he'd been on Ritalin, I'd found that sorting through baseball cards and reading were new skills that we could reward with appropriate gifts, like books. He'd come a long way from the child who'd happily ripped pages out of a Christmas book in Middletown, thinking that that was the right approach to all of that colorful, glossy paper.

"I want a brother, Mom." He threw the sentence out somewhat casually, but because there was no hesitation in his reply, it was obvious that he'd given this some thought.

I stopped our nightly prayer ritual and straightened up in surprise.

"You do? Why?"

My husband and I didn't come from big families, and we certainly hadn't been entertaining the thought of having more kids, especially in front of the children, so I was a bit taken aback.

"I don't know. I just do. We can call him Hadji."

Then, to end the discussion, he stuck his two fingers in his mouth, and turned away from me to go to sleep.

I had laughed as I returned to our bedroom to tell my husband that Haywood wanted us to expand our brood for his birthday present, and that his favorite show, "Jonny Quest," was the inspiration for this desired child's name.

"Guess what? Haywood says he wants a brother. Can you believe it? I've never heard him say anything like that."

"I always wished I'd had a brother too," my husband replied, "but that's just not in the cards for us. I don't want to take any more chances, and I know you don't want to go on and off medication again, or deal with morning sickness. What did you say to him? You didn't say yes, did you?"

"Are you kidding? I didn't say anything. I just laughed."

Now, sitting on the phone with my speechless husband, I was recalling that conversation, wondering if my son had known something before we had. Stranger things had happened in our lives.

Haywood hadn't yet made the connection between that May conversation and our July reality. He was still processing the fact that this was the second time I'd called him at work with surprise news about having a baby.

"Well, so much for birth control," he said.

"No kidding. The factory is officially closed after this one, sweetie. From now on, the ball is in your court. You're going to have to get fixed. For a woman who couldn't even have her period until her twenties, now I'm too fertile for my own good, with or without birth control."

"Let's talk about *that* another time," Haywood said, quickly changing the subject. We said our goodbyes and hung up, needing to process this new piece of information in our own private ways.

I immediately started thinking about the practicality of a third child.

For one, I didn't have a single baby item left. When we moved to Washington, I'd pared our possessions down to the essentials, and had sold everything to a second-hand store in Baltimore. Within the last six weeks, my older sister, Lizzie, had told me that she was expecting her first child and I'd given her whatever baby clothes I had left over, which wasn't much.

Secondly, all of the bedrooms in our house were taken. Haywood was in a boyish room with blue walls and Legos everywhere. Samantha was in the small bedroom next to his, and I'd just decorated it in pale green with yellow elephants marching around the middle of the wall. A baby wouldn't work particularly well in either room, plus we'd promised both children that they didn't have to share a bedroom ever again. Haywood's hyperactivity and early rising had been hard for Samantha, who was not wired to require as little sleep, so the separation created by the move had been ideal. So where would Miller Baby number 3 go?

I barely had time to contemplate these questions before my body completely shut down. Instead of just crashing off of the Wellbutrin, as I'd done when I'd learned I was pregnant with Samantha, now I had to go off two stimulants abruptly, and it was ugly. Ritalin had been studied for so many decades that I had no fear of the fetus' exposure to it, but my body had just happily acclimated to both of these medications, so going off them cold turkey sent me into an emotional and physical tailspin.

Everything changed overnight. My daily exercise of biking, running or walking was eliminated as I struggled to simply wake up and go through the basic motions of being a mother. I was incredibly lucky that my pregnancy coincided with our hosting of a young French woman, who had needed a place to live temporarily while she immersed herself in the English language. Muriel had come to us through some friends of ours, who had asked if we needed a babysitter in exchange for room and board for a few months, and although our basement "bedroom" wasn't much to speak of, Muriel had cheerfully installed herself there and didn't bat an eye when we leaned heavily on her now to help me with my kids' routines.

I didn't think I'd ever felt so awful in my entire life. My irritatingly upbeat, handsome and fit new Ob/Gyn annoyed me by saying that I was simply having another healthy pregnancy because of the worse-than-ever morning sickness. Something about the fact that he clearly didn't comprehend the magnitude of the nausea, and that men never contorted their lives and bodies like this to have children, really pissed me off, even though I knew it was totally irrational.

In a burst of immaturity and unwillingness to completely accept the fact that I was going to be a mother again, I decided to skip all of the prenatal appointments after the initial ones. I was too tired to educate another set of doctors about why I stood on the scale backwards, plus I didn't want to go through endless bloodwork and the dreaded glucose tolerance test, either. I simply banked on the fact that my child would be fine, even though I was slightly surprised that no one in the doctors' offices ever noticed that I only reappeared around the eighth month to finalize the delivery details.

My carefully constructed life of writing and mothering also took a nosedive. I was midway through a two-book contract with Prentice-Hall, and needed to turn the first one in just as my third book, a daily guide to dealing with depression, *Bright Words for Dark Days*, was about to be published by Bantam in November 1994. Between the fatigue and nausea throughout the summer months, I could barely sit and focus at my desk to do the requisite work. Samantha even picked up on my misery, and began to stand at the top of the basement stairs, pounding on the closed door and crying that she wanted to see me. "Mommy!" she would shriek, over and over again.

Something about our decision not to send Haywood to the school I'd attended as a child had also set my parents off. I didn't know if our move was seen as a repudiation of my own childhood, but I once again became a target of criticisms that came out of nowhere, and without provocation. I dressed poorly, my children were rude, and my decorating decisions were wrong. One bizarre day, I even watched my mother's feet march back and forth on my front lawn from the basement window well as she mowed the grass without asking if I wanted her to do it. Later, when I brought it up, she'd said that my neighbors were going to be offended at my slovenly approach to lawn care, so she'd taken matters into her own hands to make things right and prevent my reputation from tanking.

I felt besieged from all sides. I couldn't do anything right, it seemed. Haywood's parents freely criticized me for trying to be a working mother, noting that Haywood's sister didn't work at all, and that was a far superior approach to child-rearing. "You only think about yourself," my father-in-law said once, piercing me to the core. Hadn't they noticed my endless attempts to work from home and contribute to our income so that my children could see me as much as possible? Didn't that count for anything in their parenting books? And didn't they remember our recent bankruptcy situation? I'd hated trying to salvage Renewal with a newborn in my arms, but it had been necessary. In the absence of my own parents' compliments, my in-laws' criticisms felt particularly unkind and off-the-mark.

Haywood felt trapped between wanting to be a supportive husband and not wanting to alienate his parents by giving them ultimatums about how he expected them to treat their daughter-in-law. One of the biggest themes we returned to in our arguments over the years was that he knew that his father had created scores of enemies with this type of behavior over the years, burning bridges in every city he had lived in, and he didn't want to become one more bridge that his father burned in the process of standing up for me.

While I sympathized with his plight, it created misery for me because of my inability to find a safe place where I felt protected from their criticism of my parenting. My husband, for his part, confided often in our friends that the greatest sadness of his adult life had been how his parents had recreated the same in-law strife they'd had with their own parents—a situation they had sworn never to foist upon their own children. It was an unhappy problem that never found a solution, other than me keeping my distance, but at least I held fast to my own self-care, refusing to become a Stepford wife just to satisfy his parents' expectation of who I was supposed to be. I'd fallen for that type of pressure when I tried to be thin and perfect for my own parents, and I wasn't going to fall into that type of trap again for anyone.

The bigger and more physically vulnerable I became, the greater my mother's attacks on me and my life. She took offense and said I was "too sensitive," which was her usual comeback when I disagreed with her or asked her to temper her comments. If we were at odds, it was always because something was flawed in me—I was "too touchy," I had "no sense of humor," or I had "put a cruel spin on an innocent comment." There was never an apology; it was always just an attack on my reactions to her.

The quality of my writing was also "off" during this period because my heart just wasn't in it any longer. With Muriel departing for France right after Thanksgiving, I couldn't imagine how I was going to juggle writing another book with an infant, a two-year-old, and a five-year-old, even if I got some household help. I felt that if I continued to try to write part-time and be a mom, no one was going to get the best of me. The publisher wouldn't, my children wouldn't, my husband wouldn't, and I wouldn't. I would be pulled in too many directions.

I decided to wave the white flag of surrender. I called my agent and said I wanted to send back half of the advance so that Prentice Hall could find another writer for the second book. It was an admission of defeat. I was over my head and needed a break from work to integrate this third child into our family.

Despite my relief about easing my professional obligations, I began to feel that my emotions were steadily fraying because of my parents' peculiar and offensive behavior. Part of it, I thought, could be due to the fact that my grandmother, Donny, had become too difficult to care for at home, and my mother had decided to move her to a nursing home. Although I thought it was a good decision for Donny to receive more specialized care, I was upset that my mother chose to put her three hours away on the Delaware shore where it would be almost impossible for me to visit her as regularly as I would have liked.

My father's health was also beginning to fail noticeably. In the beginning of my pregnancy, he had called to inform me that his doctors thought he had Parkinson's disease, and he was starting some medications to try to slow its progression. He still swam regularly, went to work, and looked fit, but the lapses in his memory and his occasionally shuffling gait were give-aways that something was terribly wrong.

Even taking into account my father's gradual decline and the stress she'd felt from caring for her own mother, however, didn't completely explain the enormous hostility that my mother now directed full-force at me. Her venom reached a crescendo during a pivotal few days when *Bright Words for Dark Days* was being released. It was a busy and important week for me. Not only was a book party being held in my honor at a neighbor's house, but I was also hosting a baby shower for my sister, who was flying into town from Boston to come to my book party.

Knowing my lack of cooking skills, and the fact that my hands were full with my family duties, my mother had offered to pay for a caterer to ensure that the baby shower attendees had an impressive meal, and that my sister's party would be judged a success by all who attended. Although something inside me was wary about the offer, I decided to accept.

A few days before my sister's baby shower, the phone rang.

"Caroline, I have decided to cancel the caterer for the party." My mother's voice was eerily calm.

The fact that I was hearing this just as I was at a breaking point with my family and professional obligations made something in my frazzled brain snap.

"You're doing what?" I couldn't believe what I was hearing. This was coming out of left field, and like so many other things that had happened in my life, seemed to be fueled by my mother's bottomless desire to hurt me in some way, particularly in a moment of personal triumph. Anything that was good news for me—like the launch of a book—had always represented bad news for her.

I berated myself for letting down my guard. Why had I been stupid enough to allow my mother to pay for a caterer when this was her estab-lished lifelong pattern? I felt like Charlie Brown, hopefully running towards the football that Lucy was holding, praying that Lucy wouldn't pull it away again. But, like the Peanuts characters, I was always going to be Charlie

Brown who never got to kick the ball, and she was always going to be Lucy.

I hung up the phone and started to call every friend I had who was a good cook. I was expecting thirty people and wasn't experienced enough to know how to pull this off without significant help.

Fortunately my friends came through. A woman down the street made baked brie with a pretty leaf cut-out on top. A few others whipped up desserts and dropped them off. I bought a vat of chicken salad and plain rolls to go with it. A few of my closer friends showed up the morning of the shower to buoy my spirits, polish my silver, and vacuum. As a result, the party went off without a hitch, but I'd reached a point with my parents where I simply had to take a new and different stand. My years of therapy, unbroken recovery and growing self-confidence could not withstand the constant hostile fusillade from two blocks away.

"We need to find a family therapist," I said to my younger brother in exasperation shortly after this embarrassing occurrence. Billy was a newly-wed who lived nearby with his wife. I called him up one day with my idea for a possible family truce.

"We've never had anyone look at our family as a unit and give us feedback about how to communicate effectively with each other, and we need to do it now before it's too late. Dad's getting worse and I'm simply not going to have time to spend on trying to deal with them after the baby is born. It's now or never for me."

My brother agreed and was game to participate in this effort; my sister, who was about to deliver her baby in Boston, could not.

Now, as I tried to think of any reason to explain the non-stop anger towards me, I thought about a brother, Scott, who had sadly died within days of his birth in late 1964. Was it possible that my mother had begun to hate me after she returned empty-handed from the hospital that cold November day? Had I been such a hyperactive handful that she'd lashed out at me in her anger about Scott's death, and never got over the loss? After all, it was now the month that marked the thirty year anniversary of that occasion, and the book I had just published documented the existence of mysterious "anniversary depressions." Without people even being aware of this phenomenon, it had been shown that we fall into funks on the anniversaries of sad times in our lives, such as deaths, abortions or family tragedies. Was this what was going on? I had never entertained this thought before. Could it explain part of what was happening between us now?

I didn't have any answers, but I knew we needed professional help if we were ever going to make progress and see peace in our time. And if we didn't act quickly, our family was going to coalesce into cold and isolated camps. I didn't want this for me or my children, so I decided to put one last effort into bridging our differences. I'd done too much work in therapy not to hope that this "Hail Mary" pass might help us find some mutual love and acceptance before it was too late.

Kathleen didn't have any family therapists to recommend in our area, so Billy and I put the word out that we were looking for a skillful person who was good at negotiating tricky family landmines. We also knew that our parents had the old-fashioned view that men were more authoritative in matters like this, so we narrowed the list down to experienced male therapists who fit the bill.

Only one name came back as someone who had the background and skills to deal with us and whom my parents would respect. Eric Shepherd was a late-forties former Green Beret from Vietnam who'd earned the reputation of being unafraid to wade into conflicts and wrestle the combatants to the ground. If you just wanted to chat, he wasn't the right guy. If we wanted results in the compressed time we had available, he was the only game in town. We were told that he had top-secret government clearance, and had even worked in conflict negotiation with embassies. Only one problem: he was booked from 6 a.m. until 9 p.m. most days and had a waiting list. We decided to try, anyway, after my brother got my parents to agree to attend a few sessions before my baby was due in late February 1995.

My life as I knew it, and my recovery as I'd thought of it, was about to be drastically challenged. It would become my own Vietnam War and a fight for my life in ways I'd never contemplated before.

## CHAPTER EIGHTEEN
## BRAIN-DAMAGED

We finally got a two-hour block of time in Dr. Shepherd's Bethesda office in early 1995. On the appointed afternoon, my brother, my parents, and I gathered and made awkward small talk in his small waiting room.

If the pictures on the walls were any indication of what we were about to experience, it was going to be interesting. Instead of framed credentials and tranquil water machines, like I'd seen in Kathleen's office and the offices of countless other mental health professionals, dozens of photographs dotted the beige walls. I guessed they were scenes from Dr. Shepherd's travels to far-flung places—the pyramids of Egypt, the rainforests of South America, African plains. Pictures of snakes vied with shots of naked children in tribal settings. Even a quick glance at these images would lead someone to the conclusion that there wasn't much that Dr. Shepherd hadn't seen, done, or survived.

I was studying pictures of a long-lashed camel in front of a pyramid when Dr. Shepherd's office door swung open. The four of us turned together to look at Mr. World Traveler and got an unexpected eyeful.

Eric Shepherd was massive in both size and energy; his frame filled the entire doorway. He introduced himself to each of us with a crushing handshake. His shirt was unbuttoned enough that I could see a gold necklace and a hairy chest, and his shirtsleeves were rolled up to expose the biggest forearms I'd ever seen.

In my 33 years and my extensive travels through the self-help, therapy and hospital settings, I had never met a mental health professional who even remotely resembled Dr. Shepherd. Although a beard was a staple of many male therapists, everything else about this guy was completely unlike anything I'd seen before. His casual ensemble of jeans, a vented hiking shirt, and Hush Puppies without socks suggested that he was comfortable enough in his own skin not to care what we thought about his outfit, his pictures, or anything else. This was intriguing, particularly in a town where everyone strove to conform to the norm and where standing out meant getting shot at. That's exactly what I'd been trained to do, so I wondered what my parents thought of Dr. Shepherd's unconventional presence, but didn't dare glance at them.

We silently trooped into his office. I was already slightly off-balance because I had imagined someone a bit older and more conservative in appearance. I suddenly had no idea what this was going to be like or what to expect from this session. I caught sight of some drums on an air conditioner. Were we going to drum together to pound out our frustrations? Nothing would have surprised me at this point.

"Call me Shep," Dr. Shepherd said as he settled into a black leather chair covered with beads. My father and mother sat together on a couch under a picture of the wilds of Alaska. My brother took refuge in a recliner across the room in front of a bookcase crammed with books, globes and strange-looking statues. I perched nervously by myself on a small couch, as close to Shep as I could get. "Right Way!" told me that this was the safest place to be if I wanted some protection. I picked up a throw pillow and put it over my stomach.

I surreptitiously looked around. Feathered headdresses were bunched together on one wall, next to a variety of mounted spears and gruesome masks. I was afraid to gawk, but I also knew that I was sitting directly under a bunch of fish and mermaids that were suspended from the ceiling. This guy was a piece of work. I wondered what kind of training he'd had, but the requisite row of framed certificates was off to the left and out of my field of vision.

Shep smiled and looked around the room, taking us all in with a head-to-toes swish of his eyes. I could tell that there was probably not much he didn't catch. "So why are you all here today?"

Shep got an earful that afternoon, to say the least. As I suspected, my parents had many pent-up complaints about me, going back to when I was very young. As I listened to them talk about the ways that I hadn't measured up to their expectations, I became angry and defensive. Several times, my voice rose as I pleaded with them to see me or my life in a more generous light.

My brother joined in from time to time with his own thoughts, but it quickly degenerated into an altercation between me and my parents, with Billy's presence being almost inconsequential.

"Caroline is the problem in the family, not Billy," my parents stated again and again. "He's only here because she made him come." Really? They didn't think my brother was capable of making his own decisions?

Like every other time in my life, I was the odd man out in my family, with my brother helplessly sitting on the sidelines while he watched the team of my mother and father fire their verbal cannons at me. For an ailing man in his mid-sixties, my father did pretty well with his assaults as he talked about a variety of "problems," including an unfounded accusation that I'd purposely put a hole in the wall of their Bethany Beach home one weekend. "That's what she's like," he said, shaking his head. "We can't trust her."

"I did not!" I practically levitated from my seat in anger. I had no idea what they were talking about, but I did know that I hadn't put a hole in any wall anywhere, and I resented being blamed for something so bizarre.

"How could you possibly say something like that?" I screamed.

I was starting to feel like I was going crazy, which I'd often felt when I was younger and an accusation had been hurled at me that I couldn't possibly defend myself against.

"You said awful things about me to your friends, and that's why they looked at me strangely when I walked into the room," my mother said to me one day in fury when I was twelve. It didn't matter that she'd imagined the entire scenario; I was just helpless in the face of the rage that emerged from nowhere like a violent cloudburst whenever she became convinced that I'd done something that was wrong or reflected poorly on her. Sometimes her anger went on for days, and I was given the silent treatment whenever we were alone, but not when outsiders were around. Now I was being blamed for some hole in a wall somewhere that I knew nothing about, and I felt like my head was about to burst.

Shep spun from one argument to the next, challenging all of our perceptions of various family situations and asking us to put ourselves in each other's shoes several times. At one point he barked, "Shut up!" at me when I began to scream at my parents as they stuck to their stories that they'd been responsible, kind, loving people, and that many of the issues I was raising were fiction. "I don't recognize myself in that story," my mother said dismissively, as I recounted the caterer incident.

Shep's admonition to be quiet shocked me into compliance. No one had said anything like that to me, but he could see and feel the frustration that was overtaking me, and needed me to cool off.

After two hours, we had certainly aired our issues, but I didn't feel we were any closer to understanding or mutual respect than we'd been when we walked in. Shep asked us to commit to a total of four two-hour sessions prior to my baby's birth to see if we could make any headway. He pointed out that we'd at least listened to each other that day, even if we still disagreed. We all committed to come back two weeks later for round number 2.

The next session with Shep was similar to the first one. Once again, the session telescoped down to a "Caroline Versus Her Parents" title bout. It became increasingly clear to me, too, that the thing I was proudest of—my long-term recovery from bulimia—was the "proof" my parents used that I was a liar, and that I could not be trusted.

Instead of really seeing me for who I was today—a woman who'd had the courage to seek help for bulimia when almost nothing was known about the illness, who had gotten better, written four inspirational books, started and run a non-profit to educate others, and who continued to be free of an eating disorder—I was a major disappointment to them. Nothing I'd done in recent years mattered to my parents. Over and over again, they returned to their belief that I was a mess, and that I always would be. My eating disorder battle was the proof that I was the problem in the room today, and they were sure that Shep saw it, too. "She vomited her way through Harvard, of all places," my mother said in a disgusted, condescending tone at one point. "I can't believe she did that to us."

\* \* \* \* \* \* \* \* \*

"I CAN'T BELIEVE she did that to us." That comment haunted me during the remaining weeks of our time with Shep. I had "done" something to my parents by succumbing to bulimia, and instead of having the empathy to see that I'd been the one hurting all of those solitary years, and that their abusive actions had contributed to my condition, they said that *they* felt like the true victims. Their self-absorption, and unwillingness to see my eating disorder as anything other than an affliction they'd had to bear, was hard to accept.

I brought it up in our fourth session. It was my last chance to see if we could come to some sort of understanding on this point.

"Do you really see yourselves as the victims of my eating disorder?" I asked wonderingly one cold February afternoon. The baby in my stomach had now dropped so low that I knew childbirth couldn't be far off. A sonogram had confirmed that Haywood would be getting his wish for a brother, and I knew from his sudden lack of kicking that this boy was going to be here before long.

"You made every situation unpleasant, Caroline. Now we know some of why all of those years were so hard," my mother responded coldly. "It wasn't because of us."

My heart sank. I didn't even feel like fighting back any longer. My desire to work on family healing had been extinguished by the conversations I'd heard here during the last two months. I could see now that it had been a hopeless venture. It was obvious to me that I'd never really been loved by these two people, and that their way of justifying their ugly behavior towards me was to point out that I was simply unlovable, and a lying bulimic on top of it.

My work with Kathleen had brought me to the place where I accepted that my parents' parenting had been awful; now I understood for the first time that there had probably never been any kind of bond between them and me. Absorbing this fact as a hugely pregnant woman who loved my two children and my unborn baby more than I had ever imagined I could love anyone, felt like being trapped in a horror show.

It didn't register with them that I'd been denied affection and acceptance at every turn, nor were my parents even capable of admitting it. I didn't even bother bringing up the time my mother had informed me that she was going to drop me off at an orphanage when I was in third grade. It would be her word against mine, and she'd say it didn't happen like she denied everything else that reflected poorly on her. She'd also deny slapping me so hard one afternoon when I was making Christmas cookies at the age of eight with my sister that blood poured out of my nose for almost an hour. She wouldn't cop to the multiple times I had walked into the kitchen in the morning, only to see brochures for boarding schools on the breakfast table.

"We're sending you away. We don't want you here anymore," my dad said on several occasions by way of explanation. At other times, while I'd be studying for a test in high school, my mother would burst into my room without knocking and tell me that it didn't really matter if I studied or not—they were going to pull me out of National Cathedral any day because I didn't deserve to be there. Just like with the orphanage, these scenes had been empty, terrifying threats designed to scare me and make sure I got the message: We don't want you.

This had gone on and on, to the point where I almost didn't care whether they made good on their intentions or not. I'd taken my grief out on myself with vicious binging and purging sessions to ease the ongoing anxiety and what I now understood was probably depression, too. Because of these "we don't want you" messages that started young, the stories I read in newspapers about parental grief when children left for college seemed like fairytales. There were parents who loved their children so much that they wanted them to be around and not leave for college? Who were they? I certainly couldn't relate to that experience. When it was time to send me to Harvard, my mother had even called the university mid-summer to plead with them to take me early.

"There must be something she can do," I heard her say from her bedroom down the hall from where I sat listening. "How early can you take her?" In the end, I'd been shipped off to Harvard a few weeks early so that I could clean bathrooms and earn a little money. When my parents had actually arrived with all of my possessions, my mother made a scene at the Freshman Picnic because she perceived that I'd been rude to her.

"Everyone saw what you did," she huffed as she turned away in her familiar pique about an imaginary slight. So while everyone else was hugging their tearful parents goodbye, I was standing forlornly in the middle of Harvard Yard with no one to hug. As usual, they'd found a way to pick a fight with me during yet another supposed highlight in my life, and, once again, they'd taken the stance that it was all my fault. My whole life felt like it had been one crazy-making scene after the next that would cause anyone to doubt their sanity.

Sitting here in Shep's office seventeen years later, it was obvious that I had changed dramatically over the years, but that they had not and didn't see why they should. Their position was clear: Caroline is damaged goods. The unhelpable, unlovable one. The child who has always been nothing but trouble, and who has now dragged her poor brother here to family therapy to advance her campaign against her defenseless parents.

Couldn't Shep see what they were up against? My two bright, well-educated, attractive parents pleaded with him to take their side and help them in their fight against me.

Shep recognized exactly what was happening, but his response wasn't what they expected. In his final attempt to reach them, he tried to budge my parents from their unyielding position with a visual prop.

"This is your daughter," he noted, reaching over to a grab a tiny black woolen sheep that was perched on a table next to him. "She is the black sheep and the identified patient in this family. Do you know what that means?"

My mother, who usually withdrew into indignant silence when she wasn't accusing me of various misdeeds, merely shook her head, while my father replied, a little too calmly, "No, Dr. Shepherd. Please tell us."

"The identified patient is the person in the family who is the scapegoat, or what is often called 'the black sheep.' Caroline gets a lot of attention, rightly or wrongly, in this family for being the black sheep, and by focusing all of your energy on her, it prevents all of you from taking responsibility for your own behaviors."

Shep's voice was loud and angry. I think he was frustrated by his lack of apparent headway with the four of us, and didn't know what else to do to get my brother and parents to step up to the plate and state what their own issues were in making sure that this unbalanced dynamic remained securely in place. Too much of the eight hours had revolved around criticisms of me, and it was clear to Shep that as long as I remained the identified patient, nothing in this family was ever going to change for the better.

My father quickly changed direction. "Dr. Shepherd?" he began coolly, leaning forward to get Shep's attention. My father never called the therapist "Shep," and was usually careful to keep his pleasant demeanor on display in this office. He was a nice, hardworking guy in many settings, with many admirers and friends.

At home, however, I hadn't always seen this gentle side of him, particularly if any alcohol had been consumed, or if he had fought with my mother. I'd lost count of the times he'd locked me out of the house after our arguments, occasionally when I was just in a flimsy nightgown and it was cold outside. On miserable nights like that I would peek in the windows and wait for him to finally unlock the front door, which was my signal that it was permissible to let myself in and go to my room. These incidents were never discussed the following day, nor had I ever heard an apology for what he'd done. At times I even wondered if I'd dreamt the whole scenario because it was always business as usual, with no discussion of what was really happening.

Dad now had Shep's attention so he continued with his question.

"Caroline's mother and I have always wondered about something that happened when she was just a baby. I wonder if you could give us your professional opinion?"

In my wildest dreams, I couldn't have imagined what came out of his mouth next. We all sat there expectantly, wondering what type of professional opinion was needed about me.

"When Caroline was just an infant, we got into a car accident. Her baby seat was thrown to the floor of the car and she hit her head."

My father paused before asking the "big" question.

"Dr. Shepherd, my wife and I have always wondered if Caroline suffered brain damage from this incident, and if that is why she's always been, well... *difficult*." He concluded with a small, self-effacing laugh.

The silence in the room was almost too much to bear. My parents had just asked this therapist, Dr. Shepherd, if I, a *magna cum laude* Harvard graduate and best-selling author, might be brain-damaged. No one said anything for a moment as the question hung in the air.

"No," Shep finally said in a resolute, low voice. "That's not possible. Your daughter is not brain-damaged."

In that short exchange, several critical emotions passed through me. The first one was shock. I'd heard my parents lie about me, accuse me of hurting their possessions, disparage my battle with bulimia and berate me for being a bad mother. They'd criticized me openly, made endless fun of me and called me names I wouldn't call my enemy.

But one thing they'd never undermined was my intelligence. That was the only thing about me that had never been in dispute from the time I'd been put on the private school testing treadmill. In fact, on one occasion in my teens my father had waved my Stanford-Binet Intelligence test results at me when we'd been arguing.

"The Great White Hope," he said derisively, flashing the scores in front of my face. "The person who could have been something but never made it."

Now, instead of hearing about my high intelligence, my parents were asking a mental health professional if I was brain-damaged. I had officially fallen down the rabbit hole and felt like the Mad Hatter in *Alice in Wonderland*. The world was upside-down and I was at a tea party where everyone was nuts.

I stared at my parents with sudden, cold clarity. Now I knew why they had agreed to come here. These four sessions had simply been a campaign to convince a highly credentialed professional that they were long-suffering victims of their brain-damaged daughter. If they could get him to take their side, then they would have their proof that I'd been the problem all along, not them, and they'd never have to change or admit their shortcomings. Dr. Eric Shepherd was supposed to have been their biggest catch in a lifelong quest to vilify me.

Shep, however, had not gone along with their agenda. I felt a surge of profound gratitude, even though he had no idea how many puzzle pieces had just come together in my head. His stalwart refusal to let my parents have their way and label me as brain-damaged marked the first and only time in my life that someone had stood up for me in front of my parents and in the face of their outlandish criticisms. The approach that had worked for my parents for years had failed here. Shep had called it like he saw it, and I knew deep-down that he was right about his diagnosis: I was the "identified patient" in the family, and everyone was using my well-known struggles and admission of bulimia to avoid facing themselves or their own roles in this established family dynamic.

Dr. Eric Shepherd had just earned his fat fee in my head. He was as good as everyone had said he was, and I was grateful for the gift he'd just unknowingly bestowed upon me.

* * * * * * * *

I WAS DONE. I needed to get out of this office as fast as I could. I wanted to be around my husband and children. I needed to be enveloped in love and sanity, not hatred and craziness. This was absurd. There was never going to be harmony in this family. If everyone else didn't want it, why should I fight for it?

I turned to Shep. "That's it for me," I said with finality. "I've heard all I need to hear and there's nothing more to say. This isn't good for me, and I need to think about myself and this baby now. Thank you for your time. I do appreciate your efforts."

Our session concluded and we all left. I had no idea what anyone else took away from that final session, but I needed to get away and digest what had happened. Something profound had shifted and I felt like some of the final scales had dropped from my eyes about where I really stood with my parents, both now and for the rest of our lives.

Kathleen's comment about the Leaning Tower of Pisa came back to me as I drove home. I'd matured in many of the ways I'd dealt with my family, but now I needed to look dispassionately at the results what had happened in Shep's office. I'd been unrealistically hopeful, I saw. I'd thought that if we had a trained third-party in the room, we'd all come together and make a pact to grow as a unit. Surely, I'd thought, the pain of these strained relationships and crazy arguments was too much for my parents too, and we'd all work as a family to take responsibility for our own behaviors so that it could end.

Wrong. That wasn't the same goal that drove my parents. And now I knew it and felt a sense of relief because I wasn't going to fight for harmony and mutual understanding any longer. I wasn't going to cling to the idea that beneath the abusiveness there had been misplaced love. I wasn't going to hope for something that could never be. In the words of my self-help group, I was going to finally stop going to the hardware store for milk.

I knew that I was going to have to return to this painful topic to explore how to emotionally unhook from my parents' behaviors once and for all, particularly because I was planning to remain in the neighborhood. I would have to learn how to handle the insanity of their unpredictability without becoming unhinged or dragging my children into the vortex. I guess that meant I was going to have to go back into therapy again to find out how much more was waiting for me to explore. Happiness was, indeed, an inside job, and it appeared I'd have to go a bit deeper than I'd thought to find it when it came to family of origin issues.

But that would have to wait for just a bit. It was time to turn my attention to having a baby and using all of my energies and thoughts to make this as joyful an arrival as possible.

## CHAPTER NINETEEN
## TIME TO FLY

Bayard Rule Miller, a fifth-generation Washingtonian, came quietly into the world late on the night of February 25th, 1995 at George Washington University Hospital. Because I was sick at the time of delivery, Bayard, another near-ten-pounder, was yellow with jaundice and under the weather himself, so we had to treat him like a plant and expose him to sunlight in front of a window to return him to health.

When we brought Bayard home from the hospital, we were just putting the finishing touches on the addition we'd decided was necessary to make the house more compatible for a five-person family. Our roof had been raised, a wall had been knocked out, and an open-air stairway now wound its way up to the finished third floor containing a bedroom for Haywood, a new bathroom, and an office for me. Eventually, I knew, I'd return to some sort of work, and this home office would be the perfect spot when that time came. It was peaceful up there, with a glorious beech tree right outside my window, and skylights above.

My new mission was clear: I needed to integrate Bayard into the family, which wouldn't be so hard in the absence of trying to meet writing deadlines. I also needed to carve out a very different relationship with my parents that didn't exclude them from my children's lives, but that protected me from their behavior. I took long walks with Bayard and Samantha in a double stroller on a trail near our home as I contemplated this necessary and complicated shift.

It was going to be tricky, particularly because my father had become progressively worse since our sessions with Shep, and the doctors now thought his diagnosis was far more serious than they'd originally thought. How could I walk the tightrope of taking care of myself and my children, while also being as responsive as possible to my dying father? Even though I didn't agree with how my parents felt about me, and I hated the things they'd done to me, it wasn't in me to completely turn my back on my father.

I finally decided to call Shep that summer to see if he'd work with me on an individual basis while I sorted through these dilemmas. Returning to Shep's office by myself felt like revisiting a battlefield of fallen soldiers. I told him so as I took my place on the couch.

"That's a good analogy," he said as he settled into the black chair with beads. "I could see when we met that you would have to grieve the death of your illusions about your parents and whatever you thought they could give to you. If you really want to separate from them and own the fact that you are a black sheep, you have a lot of years of therapy ahead of you."

"How many?"

"A lot," he repeated, nodding decisively. "You have to be effectively re-parented because you were never parented in a loving way, and then you need to separate in a healthy manner. That's going to take some time, and it's not going to be easy."

Why was I the one sitting here, planning to start another round of expensive therapy? Why wasn't anyone else in my family doing it? Didn't that mean I was the one who had problems?

"On the contrary," Shep responded, "the black sheep is often the healthiest one in the family because he or she has the courage to speak the truth when others don't, and that's often why they become the black sheep in the first place. When you say something that no one wants to hear, you aren't going to win any popularity contests, and you certainly haven't won any within your family."

What Shep said about acknowledging unpopular truths really hit home because I was still holding onto some of the worst ones, and I realized that in order for me to fully heal, it was time for them to face them and let them completely come to light.

The main issue I was hiding was that I'd been physically abused for years by my father, and I'd never talked to anyone about it in depth, although I glossed over bits and pieces of those years in my two previous therapy stints. My mother had hit me, too, but less often. I decided to share some of the worst stories with Shep now so that he'd have a fresh context within which to begin our individual work.

In a scene that had played out over and over, increasingly during my teens, my father would arrive home from his day at work and my mother would tell him that I deserved to be punished for any variety of infractions or imaginary slights. I'd hear the low murmuring in the kitchen and the clink of the martini glass as they discussed their terrible daughter. I'd hold my breath, knowing full well what was about to happen, and it always did.

The scenes were ugly. At first I'd cry when the hitting started while my mother watched from the open door of my bedroom. I'd beg him to stop. I'd pray for intervention from someone, anyone. That never happened, and no one ever came to my rescue. My sister didn't want any part of it, lest she'd become the target, and my brother was simply too young at that time to do anything.

I learned to be stoic, but sometimes it just made things worse because they needed to see me suffer for the beating and kicking to stop.

My father was careful to never leave visible marks. No one could possibly know what happened in this perfect home of high achievers, and my parents were confident that I'd never tell on them—which I didn't—so the cycle was perpetuated for years. Who would I tell, anyway? My grandmother knew what was happening but was powerless to do anything except pray for me when I showed up at her door, and then call my parents to tell them I was there and safe. Although she'd had the courage to leave her own husband when my mother was very small because of his alcoholism and tendency to hit her when drinking, she didn't dare stand up to her daughter lest she lose all connection with her grandchildren.

Part of the reason why I'd decided to marry so young was because it was one of the only sure ways I had to escape the beatings. The last time my father hit me was the night before I got married. The trigger had been my reaction to my parents' decision that I wasn't going to be permitted to attend my own wedding. The reason for this drastic punishment? They didn't like where Haywood's parents had chosen to hold the rehearsal dinner, and *that* was my fault, too. They were going to make me pay for it by not allowing me to show up and marry their son the following day.

The way that scene had unfolded was surreal. My father and mother called me down to the kitchen on the night of June 17th, 1983. They said they had something to tell me. I stood rooted in place before them, not knowing what was coming, but the dinner table showed signs of drinking, which meant that this wasn't going to be good.

"We're not letting you to go your wedding tomorrow," my father announced. "It was unbelievably rude of the Millers to hold the rehearsal dinner in Annapolis, and to make all of our guests drive an hour from Washington to attend it. And on top of that, our car broke down on the way home, which wouldn't have happened if the dinner had been in Washington."

That was their reason for telling me I couldn't attend my own wedding? Because my father-in-law, a Naval Academy graduate, had wanted to have our rehearsal dinner at the Naval Academy Officer's Club? They had to be kidding. It was my in-laws' right to hold a dinner anywhere they wanted, and I had thought it was nice, even though the car breakdown on the way home had come at an unfortunate moment. My mother had glared in fury at me as my father changed the tire on the side of the Washington, D.C. beltway. I'd known that this was going to come back to hurt me somehow, but certainly not like this. This was unprecedented.

Hearing that my parents were planning to bar me from going to my own wedding brought years of fury about their irrational and mean behavior to the surface. I started to scream at the top of my lungs, crying hysterically at the same time. I had nothing of substance to say, so sounds of unnatural keening took the place of whatever words might have come out of my mouth. What does a woman say when she's told she can't attend her wedding, anyway? Okay—no problem?

After furiously tossing a chair across the kitchen and yanking the door of the refrigerator open so hard that eggs flew out of the side shelf, I ran back up to my bedroom and collapsed on the ground, sobbing so hard that I thought my body would split in half. At that moment, my father entered the room, walked over to my heaving body, and hit my back as hard as he could.

"Calm down," he ordered. "We have decided that you can go." Just like my mother's stated intention to drop me off at an orphanage fourteen years earlier had only ended when I was broken and pitiful, prostrate on the floor, gripping her ankles and begging for another chance to be the daughter she wanted, my parents needed to extract one more measure of cruelty, followed by apparent kindness, before I'd be permitted to go out and live my own life. Their game was a sophisticated form of torture similar to how prisoners of war are turned into traitors. Once a prisoner's spirit is broken he has no choice except to decide that his captors are actually good people—especially if they want to salvage their own life.

I told Shep that these memories needed to be dealt with. They were now tormenting me because I'd never really allowed them to surface in their entirety, and something about the family therapy scenes had unleashed them full-force. It couldn't have come at a more complicated time, though. Every time I saw my impotent father shuffling across a room, or I heard my siblings voice their sorrow about his diagnosis—which was Shy-Drager, a deadly neurological condition that was beginning to claim him quickly—I felt nothing but contempt. I wanted an apology for those years of mental and physical abuse. I wanted some recognition of the pain he'd caused me before he couldn't communicate any longer. I even wanted to hurt him at a time when he was helpless, which sickened me. I didn't want to have these feelings or to be this vengeful person, and I didn't want my children to grow up with the bitter mother I was turning into. I needed help.

Shep listened quietly and stroked his beard thoughtfully as the stories emerged in their gruesome detail. Nothing seemed to faze him. That gave me some comfort. I needed someone much stronger than I was to help me deal with whatever was about to come up, and that time was now. We went to work.

* * * * * * * *

Being Shep's client was unlike any other therapeutic experience I'd ever had. He held fast to some important boundaries so that I could learn how to create better ones in my own life. For example, if I was late because of a childcare situation, the appointment was never extended to compensate. If it was snowing and I couldn't get to the office, I was charged the full rate because Shep had gotten there, and my not having a four-wheel drive car to navigate slippery hills in blizzards wasn't his fault. Once I showed up snuffling, and he cut short the appointment and ordered me to see a doctor, stating that I hadn't learned to take care of myself, and that he expected me to go to the walk-in clinic across the street and call him later to tell him I'd done so.

Learning better self-care and safe boundaries coincided with my father's rapid slide into a form of dementia. Although he had moments when he was lucid, he increasingly didn't know where he was, or he collapsed to the ground because his heart rate had plunged so low that he lost consciousness. On a number of occasions, Haywood and I were summoned to help my mother with some aspect of my father's care, like picking him up off the floor.

Every time I saw an ambulance speed down my street I knew they were going to rescue my father. Sometimes I could go over to help, and sometimes I couldn't because my own children needed attention, were sick, or I had other obligations. Working with Shep meant that I was better able to withstand the anger that came my way whenever I didn't jump when my mother called.

"If a mother can't take care of herself and set boundaries, my experience is that she goes down the tubes and the children go right behind her," Shep noted one day as I discussed the endless pull between attending to an infant and two other children while knowing that my father was dying two blocks away. Bolstered by these reminders, I would return home to juggle the best I could without being guilt-tripped into behavior that didn't serve me or my own family well.

My father was finally deemed too ill to remain at home and my mother put him in a nearby nursing facility. The decline in his condition was so swift that he often didn't know who I was when I went to see him. On the rare occasions when he recognized me, he spoke gibberish mixed in with my name. Sometimes, he didn't rouse himself at all during my visits, and I would sit in silence and crochet. While we took our family for a brief vacation on the Delaware shore to enjoy the beach and spend time with my grandmother, his face and body changed so drastically that I had to get onto my hands and knees to look up at him and make sure it was actually my father. It was a pathetic and cruel disease, and its ravages were making my own situation sadder by the day.

I found myself unable to hold on to my anger as I went through this shift in roles. My father was clearly diminished from a mental standpoint, and an apology to me simply wasn't in the cards. I had to work on forgiveness, instead, so that's where I put my energies with Shep on top of simply letting these long-held secrets come to the surface. Although I didn't know much about my father's parents, who had both died before my birth, I began to wonder if they'd been distant parents to my father, which had left him incapable of love. In the pictures I'd seen from his childhood, my dad was often alone, with a sad look on his face. My grandparents, who had died before he'd married my mother, had been in their forties when my dad was born, and they'd shipped him off to a military boarding school when he'd burned down an abandoned shack on a golf course. Is that where he'd gotten the idea to send me off to boarding school? Had he taken his anger out on me instead of his own parents?

* * * * * * * *

ON WHAT TURNED OUT to be my last visit to the nursing home, my father was unexpectedly lucid. His bright blue eyes fastened on me.

"I knocked you around too much, Caroline," he said simply and without preamble.

I sat down without responding. Was this the apology I'd been waiting for? Why was he acknowledging his behavior today? Was he asking me for forgiveness?

"My father says that when it's your time, it's your time," he continued, gesturing to an empty corner of the room.

I glanced over at the corner to reassure myself that no one was actually standing there, although my father's eyes remained riveted on the empty space, as if someone really was there. Although my grandfather had never met or held any of his grandchildren, I had the eerie sensation that he was actually in the room with us, and that I had just "met" him for the first time.

At that moment, a nurse came in to check on my father and take his vital signs.

"I want her to leave," my father instructed in a firm voice pointing at me. He hadn't had that type of strength in months.

She looked at me apologetically.

"I think you should leave, dear. He's having a bad day."

Actually, he was having a very *good* day, I thought to myself as I gathered my belongings and left. My dad appeared to be more alive than he'd been in a long time, and he'd clearly known who I was today, which was a change.

Driving out of the parking lot, I realized that I couldn't go home just yet. I changed direction and called my husband. "I'm heading to the mall, although I'm not sure what I'm going to do there. I'm okay. I just need to sit for a while and not do anything for anyone." He understood and told me to take my time.

I only had enough energy to sit in the atrium of the local mall and sip coffee for two hours. Wordlessly, I watched people walk by as I thought about my father and what he'd said about knocking me around too much. It felt like he had not only apologized to me in his own way, but that he'd also just said goodbye to me.

My mind began to play a Super 8 film reel of moments from my life. I remembered my dad playing the ukulele and singing, "Five Foot Two, Eyes of Blue," to me while I giggled and danced. I remembered the hundreds of times he'd refereed at swim meets and cheered me on to victory. I recalled that he'd come to a heralded piano performance I'd given in the Cathedral before the entire school in tenth grade, even though my mother had refused to come with him and honor me. He hadn't been all bad. I let the good memories wash over me until I had nothing more to replay in my head and tears were trickling down my face.

I finished my coffee and remained frozen in my seat until my brain was too exhausted to process anything else. I drove home tired, drained and feeling much older than when I'd woken up that morning. At midnight, the phone rang. I knew without even answering it that my father was dead. I picked up the receiver and my brother instructed me to go to Shady Grove Hospital, which was about twenty minutes away. He didn't say anything else; he didn't have to.

When I arrived at the hospital, my mother and brother were in the Emergency Room in a side vestibule that was surprisingly quiet and unhurried. My father lay on a table in front of me. Because there were no doctors bustling about, and no beeping machines hooked up to his body, it confirmed my suspicions. My dad was gone.

I'd never seen a dead body, so I didn't know what to do. I gingerly moved towards my father and stared at the only thing I could focus on: his hair. Although he was 69, my dad had died with a full head of blond hair. I made myself look at his upside-down face. He looked handsome and youthful in repose.

Only one thought went through my mind as I stared numbly at the man who had sung to me and hurt me. Despite decades of hearing him say that he wanted to retrace Odysseus' voyage some day, and reading count-less books about Greek myths, he'd never gone after the one thing he'd said would bring him joy.

I murmured this thought aloud with my brother and mother standing nearby.

"I know," my mother sniffled through her tears. "That was my first thought, too."

Looking at this tear-stained, disheveled woman standing in front of me made me suddenly feel very sorry for her. I knew it wasn't easy to nurse someone through a debilitating disease and death, and she'd stood by my father the whole time. At that moment she wasn't the monster who caused me so much pain; she was a grieving widow who didn't know what the rest of her life would hold.

I looked back down at my father and said, "Bye, Dad." I couldn't bring myself to kiss him, but I touched his forehead and turned away.

I stayed at the hospital for another hour while my mother arranged for my dad's body to be transferred to a mortuary. My brother offered to take her home so I left and drove home, alone. Later, I discovered that my dad had died just one day before his own father had passed away thirty-nine years earlier, and at the exact same age. The grandfather I'd never known had undoubtedly come to get his only child to take him out of his misery, and I was glad. I now knew beyond a shadow of a doubt that they'd been conversing that morning and that it had, indeed, been my dad's "time."

I called Shep as I pulled out of Shady Grove's parking lot.

"My dad just died, and I thought you should know," I said to his answering machine. "I've never seen a dead body, and I think I'm in shock." I knew he'd seen dozens and dozens of dead bodies in his life, so I picked something I knew he'd be able to help me with. I simply couldn't think of anything else to say, so I hung up.

My drive home was slow and quiet. I didn't want to get home too quickly, nor did I want to listen to any chatter on the radio. I didn't cry. I wasn't even particularly sad. In fact, the only word that came into my mind was "relieved." I actually felt better, and it surprised me. My entire life had been overshadowed by this team, my mother and father, who had worked together to try to prevent me from ever completely growing up and separating from them. Now it had been broken up forever. They couldn't hurt me anymore.

I experienced a new and strange sense of safety that I'd never felt before, and a lightness of spirit descended upon me. I was free. I was really free. It was time to fly. And that's exactly what I intended to do.

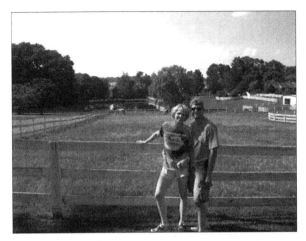

IN THE SUMMER OF 2011, HAYWOOD AND I STOPPED BY
THE FARMETTE IN BORING, MD TO SEE IF ANYTHING
HAD CHANGED, BUT IT LOOKED THE SAME
AS WHEN WE LEFT IT IN 1989.

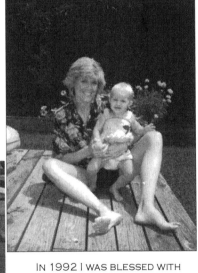

IN 1992 I WAS BLESSED WITH
SAMANTHA, WHO WAS LEARNING
TO STAND WHEN WE VISITED
BETHANY BEACH, DE, IN THE
SUMMER OF 1993.

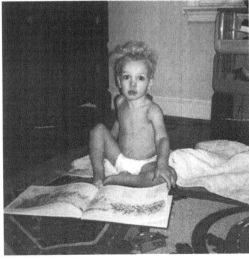

BAYARD READING AT AGE ONE

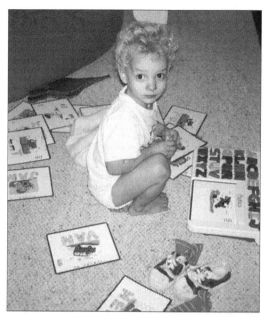

BAYARD'S FASCINATION WITH LETTERS
TOOK A PECULIAR TURN BEFORE HE
WAS TWO, LEADING US INTO A STRANGE
WORLD OF ENERGY HEALERS AND
PSYCHOLOGISTS.

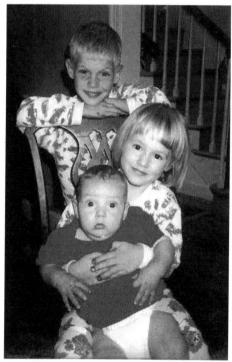

IN 1995, HAYWOOD, SAMANTHA AND BAYARD
POSED AT BEDTIME IN THEIR PAJAMAS. EVERY
PICTURE OF BAYARD IN THE FIRST YEAR OF HIS
LIFE DISPLAYED HIS WIDE-EYED ANXIETY.

170

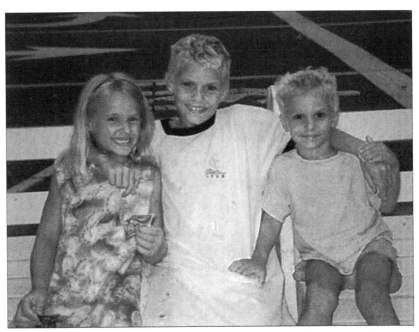

OUR THREE CHILDREN HAVE ALWAYS FOUND FRIENDSHIP AND COMFORT IN EACH OTHER'S COMPANY STARTING VERY YOUNG. IN 1997 THEY POSED ON A BETHANY BEACH BENCH BEFORE A FUN NIGHT ON THE BOARDWALK.

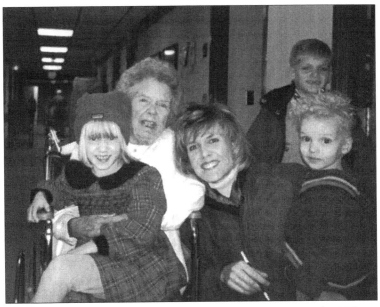

I VISITED MY GRANDMOTHER, DONNY, AT A NURSING HOME IN LEWES, DELAWARE, AS OFTEN AS POSSIBLE. ON THANKSGIVING 1996, WE ALL WENT TO SEE HER TO SHARE THE HOLIDAY.

## CHAPTER TWENTY
## BLOOD IS NOT THICKER THAN WATER

A baby bird is only ready to take flight after its mother has fed, protected and nurtured it sufficiently so it will have a fighting chance for survival. With a lot of mixed messages and negative feedback in my family nest, however, I hadn't become that baby bird capable of long-term survival. Although I'd clearly gathered enormous amounts of recovery, wisdom and strength since leaving for college and getting married, moving back to my hometown in close proximity to my parents had revealed some of the areas that still needed to be attended to. It showed me that while I no longer had an active eating disorder, I still had a way to go in terms of putting my childhood into a container so that it could cause me no further pain or, worse, negatively infect my own parenting or cause me to behave in self-destructive ways.

Shep said something one day that flew in the face of the conventional wisdom often bandied about around the importance of one's biological relatives. "Blood is not thicker than water," he stated in response to my expressed feeling of sadness about not having a strong, cohesive family to fall back on in hard times. I still found myself envious of friends who anticipated and attended warm family celebrations or participated in longstanding multi-generational rituals at summer beach homes or other familiar gathering places. Nothing like that had ever occurred in my family, nor was it likely to, and it was hard not to long for that emotional embrace that clearly gives so many people a bedrock of confidence and love.

Shep's observation came at the right moment. Just as I was trying to be patient, loving and consistent, I found myself using Shep and my godmother, Pat Griffith, to reparent *me*, just as Shep predicted I'd need. His point was accurate: I was successfully creating my own supportive family of choice and not one drop of family blood was being used.

"Aunt Pat" had always been in my life in one way or another, and had actually been one of the first people who held me when I came home from the hospital. Smart, practical and talented, she had raised two children while juggling a prestigious journalism career that took her all over the country. At the end of her writing days, which coincided with our return to my hometown, she was the Washington, D.C., bureau chief of a major newspaper chain, covering the White House, and had become one of the only women invited to join the historic and selective Gridiron Club, where journalists famously feted the President and dozens of Washington luminaries with clever skits and songs, many of which Pat wrote.

Not only was she a role model who also cared enough about me to tell me the truth when I needed it, but she had a solid and dependable Christian faith, which I longed for. She knew I'd been fighting the "stray dog" religious feelings for years, never believing that I belonged in any spiritual dwelling, so she invited me to join her on Sunday mornings when she attended a local Episcopal church. It felt nice to attend a service with someone who was so secure in her relationship with God, and I wanted some of what she had—much as I had wanted to be like the people in recovery at my early 12-step eating disorder meetings—so I signed up for some initiation classes to learn more about how to actually join the faith.

To my chagrin, I was told that I couldn't be a full participant in the church until I was baptized, which could only occur in a public service in front of the congregation. I was embarrassed that I had never been initiated into a religious faith as a child, and the idea of advertising this deficiency in front of throngs of people wasn't appealing. I didn't have a choice because they refused to do it privately, so I arranged to be baptized one Sunday morning, along with all three children not long after Bayard was born. My husband had been baptized as a baby, so his role was simply to observe and cheer us on from the pews. Pat, naturally, became the godmother to all of us, and I knew I'd finally found that safe "home."

Pat's devotion to my children was immediate and loving; they each got her individual attention, and she also gave them thoughtful gifts that spoke to their individual strengths. As they grew older, she spent hours selecting and reading books she thought they would enjoy, always inscribing them with carefully-chosen lines of wisdom and guidance. Her gesture reminded me of one of my favorite childhood memories around books. On a cross-country trip when I was in fourth grade, we had stopped in Carmel, California, to see Pat and her family. Her reverence for the importance of reading was underscored by her offer to buy my sister and me any book we wanted in a local bookstore; I chose *Little Women*. I read and reread that book throughout my childhood, thinking about Pat every time I did so. I became convinced that her support of books and the power of good writing had influenced my later decisions to write for school newspapers and pursue careers in journalism and writing books (my mother had also been an excellent writer and journalist, so I had no doubt that some of my interests were inherited from her, too). It made sense that Pat would return to my life at this particular time as a godmother, particularly because she would have been the natural choice thirty-plus years earlier if my parents had taken that step.

Shep fulfilled the other part of this "parenting" duet, encouraging, challenging and praising me for the different ways I was beginning to take risks and spread my emotional wings. One of the things I took up after Bayard's birth was rollerblading, which I'd first seen when I was waddling around Miami Beach, hugely pregnant with Bayard, while visiting my in-laws. I was taking my normal morning walk when a woman, about ten years older than me, whooshed by me in a sports bra, shorts and braids and not much else. When she turned around and sailed back towards me, the most noticeable thing was the big smile on her face. She looked completely contented, but also unimpeded by anything that could hold her back—clothes, a bad mood, or the slow gait, we mere mortals had without wheels.

I suddenly wanted to know what she felt like on those skates. What was it like to move so fast, and feel so balletic, with the self-confidence to wear only enough clothes to feel air on her stomach? I'd never had the courage to wear anything that revealing in public. Even my adult choice of bathing suits harkened back to my competition years; a one-piece Speedo was my trusted beach outfit. I wondered if I'd ever be bold enough to bare that protective skin in public.

Within a week after giving birth to Bayard, I found myself at a used sporting goods store, buying a pair of rollerblades and pads so that I could try this new sport. As I suspected, it was love at first slide. I had always loved ice skating, something my grandmother had often taken me to do, so I was immediately comfortable and able to adjust to the challenges of being on pavement instead of ice. It wasn't long before I could slip away if I had a free hour and cover eight miles down to Georgetown in Washington, D.C., and then back another eight miles for a satisfying 90-minute session. The route was particularly beautiful, starting in the heart of Bethesda on a swanky street boasting coffee stores and yoga clothing boutiques, and winding along the Potomac River until merging with the traffic near Georgetown University. Now I finally had a new outlet for my physical energy that had mostly been satisfied for years by running up and down stairs with babies strapped on my body, or pushing a double stroller along the same path I now used for my rollerblade fun.

Because of the habits I had instilled and reinforced in recovery around healthy eating and not living by the scale, I didn't have any significant weight issues to grapple with after my pregnancies. I exercised for the sheer enjoyment it provided, and not because I was trying to burn off calories in pursuit of a thin image.

After Haywood's birth, I'd learned the lesson of getting too thin without realizing that my hunger cues were off-target, but my two other pregnancies had also resulted in huge, nearly ten-pound babies without my either overeating or starving myself to get back into my clothes. I never stopped being grateful that my body was working after so many years of amenorrhea and abuse, and every time I simply returned to the same consistent size of clothing, I breathed a sigh of relief and thanked God for allowing me to continue to walk the walk, one day at a time, to this healthy place with my body where food nurtured me and exercise was a choice, not an obligation.

* * * * * * * *

JUST AS I PULLED together my family of choice and found a spiritual home, I lost one of the only people who had ever made me feel special or loved, just for being me. On the night of September 16th, 1997, I had a dark dream where I saw myself in my grandmother's room at her nursing home in Lewes, Delaware. I was floating near the ceiling in the dream, and I saw a curtain being pulled around my grandmother's bed. I didn't see her body or any other figures; all I saw was the curtain sliding with finality, and then the dream was over.

When I woke up, I couldn't shake the gloomy feelings, so I got on my bicycle to ride to and from Georgetown in an attempt to clear my head. The same path I used for rollerblading was accessible at the bottom of our street, so I made a quick trip to see if I would feel better when I got back.

As I walked back into our home and sat on the hallway steps, gathering my energy, Haywood came out of the kitchen. His face said it all.

"I'm so sorry C," he began. But before he could say another word I put my face into my hands and started to sob. I knew it was bad news about Donny. The dream had foretold her death, and he was about to confirm it.

"Donny died last night. I wish I had a better way to tell you." He hugged me and let me cry for as long as I needed to, while I processed my grief. In my most recent visit to her, she had been very together mentally, and never forgot who I was or who my children were, but she had seemed troubled as I sat on her bed to say goodbye at the end of the visit.

"I just haven't figured out what this is all about," she said, shaking her head in disappointment and sadness.

"What do you mean?" I hated to see my grandmother sad. She had

176

always been the upbeat one in my life, finding things to be positive about, and changing any conversation that wasn't about good things.

"Why we're here. Why I lived my life. What it all meant. It's just a big puzzle," she said in resignation, hanging her head. I couldn't soothe her as much as I wanted to, so I had worried on the three-hour drive home about whether or not I was visiting often enough to help keep her spirits up. My mother had put her, against our wishes, in a nursing home near the beach in a quiet town. I always wondered if she'd done it to simply wash her hands of dealing with her own mother, as well as to make it hard for the people who loved her to visit. I couldn't prove it, but it fit her pattern of being unnecessarily mean and making sure that she robbed happiness from others in any situation where she had control.

Now it was too late. Had I told Donny often enough how much I loved her? Did she really know the impact she'd had on my life and how much she mattered to me? I hoped so. She had died just two days after my 36th birthday, so maybe she was trying to let me know something by leaving at that time.

My grandmother's ashes were scattered in the Indian River inlet just north of Bethany Beach, a place she loved. At the last second before our outdoor service, I asked the crematorium to set aside a small bag of her ashes that I could keep. I didn't have anything else of hers, and didn't want to let her go completely. The little red velvet bag now sits on my bedside table, and is the first thing I see in the morning and the last thing I see when I turn out the light at night.

Why didn't my grandmother feel that she knew why she'd lived, or what she had accomplished in her 92 years? Was this something everyone felt at the very end? Was that what awaited me? I hoped not, and began to wonder if I'd be able to solve this for myself through the work I was now doing on myself.

✳ ✳ ✳ ✳ ✳ ✳ ✳ ✳

JUST AS THE sonogram had predicted when she was *in utero*, Samantha was sprouting fast and looked like she was going to pass my 5'10" height if her growth continued at the pace we were witnessing. Wherever she went, from gymnastics to music lessons to pre-school, she was always the tallest one there. The comments reminded me of my childhood. "She's so tall!" and "She's so big! How old is she?" we'd be asked. Once a stewardess had refused to let us board a flight to Florida without paying for another seat for her, despite the fact that she was still old enough to sit on our laps and travel for free.

"Ma'am," a petite woman in a blue uniform said sternly, "there is no way that child is under two years old."

We didn't have a birth certificate with us, so we bought another seat simply to get off the ground, but a sympathetic woman who overheard this dialogue took us aside and counseled us to only travel with Samantha wearing a t-shirt featuring a screen shot of her birth certificate.

"My sister's daughter faced the same problem," she confided in a low voice, "and they decided that whenever they traveled, she had to wear that shirt in case they were challenged about her age." We didn't take this step because Samantha was going to be aging out of that free flying benefit soon, but I thought it was a brilliant solution to a problem that many parents of tall children undoubtedly grappled with.

With two ex-jocks as parents, it was inevitable that we'd want our children to try athletics to see if they had any talent they wanted to pursue. We also believed that having a strong body, with the discipline that comes from being a competitive athlete, was an essential approach to a flourishing life. I recognized that while my swimming career and emphasis on wanting to look thin in a bathing suit had played a role in the development of an eating disorder, it was equally true that I'd learned how to work hard, get up when knocked down, and delay gratification in pursuit of a long-term goal from that sport. Haywood and I had also found that having a full academic and athletic life had been better than having too little to do, and that we had

178

become better organized and more productive as adults because of it.

While it was easy for our son, Haywood, to find outlets for his energy and do well on baseball, wrestling and soccer teams, Samantha hadn't shown any aptitude for anything athletic. On her kindergarten softball team, she'd been designated "pitcher's helper" to try to keep her engaged in the game, but she often studied the inside of her hat instead of following the ball. In soccer, we saw her picking flowers during one game, and one memorable morning she stuck her hands through the bottom of her shorts and with a big smile to the sidelines, yelled "Look at me!"

It was Shep who solved our concerns about Samantha growing into her body, coming up with a way to exercise and enjoy the process. "Why not try the martial arts?" he offered one day. "It's wonderful for girls, and it would be good if you did it, too, because children whose parents do the martial arts with them tend to stick with it."

It was one thing to talk about the martial arts for Samantha, but me? I could honestly say that I'd never once longed to achieve a black belt in any martial art, partly because I didn't know anyone other than Shep who had a black belt, although I had immense respect for the discipline and years of work that went into achieving that goal.

With his track record of good ideas for growth and challenge, though, I immediately started to look into the martial arts. Several people encouraged us to look at a Korean martial art called Hapkido, described as "usable self-defense," and something that many pro athletes and Secret Service agents are proficient in. Samantha and I went to two studios, both Hapkido schools, and we happened to arrive as a children's class was starting at the second one.

"She can just jump in and try it," one of the instructors said after meeting us. I didn't know exactly what to expect, so I just settled into a row of folding chairs to observe as my five-year-old daughter tried something completely alien to her life.

For an hour, Samantha kicked, bowed, punched, jumped and yelled "Yes, sir!" to every question she was asked. Although she'd never been required to answer anyone that way, she was yelling "Yes, sir!" like a pro by the end of class. After she was dismissed, she scampered back to me and with a flushed face said, "I want to do this!" The excitement in her face and her eagerness to try something so new to her sold me immediately. We'd found something that would keep her motivated and using her body in a vigorous way, with clearly designated steps for moving towards a great goal.

But what about me? I'd liked what I'd seen, but punching and kicking were two things I hadn't done since my sister and I had gotten into a fistfight as children, so that would definitely be out of my comfort zone, as would yelling, "Yes, sir!" throughout a class. What appealed to me, though, was that it looked physically challenging, and that was something I hadn't really felt in an extended way since my years of competitive swimming had ended fifteen years ago.

Two days later I went in to try a class for adults at noon, where I met a cello player, two policemen, an executive from Marriott, and several other men and women who were wearing baggy white uniforms encircled at the waist by belts ranging in color from yellow to white to brown. The instructor was a diminutive Korean young man who quickly took charge and put us through our rigorous paces. We stretched, kicked x-ray paper, performed self-defense moves, and then sparred. We ended with a short meditation, bowed to the U.S. and Korean flags, and returned to our locker rooms.

I felt the way Samantha had felt—this was cool stuff. And if my participation would be helpful to her in any way, it was more than worth it, so I signed a sheaf of forms committing us both through the red belt level, regardless of how long it would take to complete. I knew that doing this would create financial accountability that would make it tough to back out, and I wanted to remove all ambivalence about setting out on this long path.

Samantha and I became an inseparable mother-daughter duo in pursuit of a set of our belts and stripes, going twice a week at night, plus Saturday mornings, for our classes, which were usually back-to-back. The juggling of babysitters and logistics to make sure Haywood and Bayard were safely cared for during these times was a challenge, but the payoff of seeing Samantha master an intricate set of forms, kicks and new moves, and the confidence it brought her, was indescribable.

I also had an unexpected reaction to Hapkido that touched a part of me that had never quite found the necessary emotional healing. There were many positive parts of the sport that I immediately benefitted from. They included wearing shapeless uniforms that discouraged the idea of comparing body types in the ever-present mirrors. I loved the endless repetition of self-defense moves and form sequences that imprinted on my brain and eventually made the correct behavior automatic. The sequence of pre-determined behaviors reminded me of my eating disorder recovery, which also consisted of doing a lot of little things correctly, over and over, in order for the long-term outcome to be what I wanted.

Being able to do flips in the air, and learn how to fall correctly without breaking bones, was also a lot of fun, as well as useful because of my occasional spills on rollerblades. In addition, I learned a great approach to the mindset of success when we had our first board-breaking seminar. My hand bounced helplessly off the pine boards and was beginning to throb when our grandmaster came over to observe me. After watching my efforts for a minute, he stopped me and said, "Watch." Then he effortlessly swung his right hand, palm up, through the board as if it were butter. The two halves clattered to the ground.

"What's the secret?" I asked, planting my hands on my hips, frustrated that I wasn't getting it.

"Don't look at the board when you are trying to break it. Look two inches past the board where your hand strikes it, as if it has already gone through. If you just stare at the board, you will always be looking at the obstacle, not the outcome," he explained.

The wisdom in those few short sentences made sense to me on every level. I was fixated on the thing I was trying to overcome instead of seeing the victorious outcome. With that advice, my hand flew through the board, delivering a satisfying "thwack." The stack of boards I brought home as souvenirs of elbow, hand and foot-breaking was impressive to me in more ways than one because every break reinforced the wisdom of looking at where I want to go in life, not at what stands in my way.

The most surprisingly beneficial outcome of the martial arts for me, though, came during a normal noon class for adults, which I occasionally had the freedom to attend, after we had completed our routine set of self-defense moves and throws. "Get on your sparring gear!" the instructor ordered.

Although already exhausted, I strapped on my chest guard, sparring mitts, and helmet, put in my mouth guard, and returned to the mat. That day I was paired against a well-built, dark-haired cop whose behavior in the studio had earned him the moniker "Crazy Kevin." Kevin was known to take things a little too far in sparring matches and belt tests, occasionally hurting his opponents unnecessarily with an errant backhand to the head, or a too-tight grip on a chokehold. Kevin also wasn't thought to be woman-friendly, something that crossed my mind as we bowed to each other and faced off for a three-minute match.

I kept my eyes on Kevin, who was slightly shorter than me, as he began to smile and exhort me to try to get him as we cautiously bobbed around each other. "You can't hurt me," he encouraged. "Just go for it."

Was Crazy Kevin taunting me? I didn't like the way he was looking at me, so did a quick punch followed by a round kick that landed squarely on his abdomen. Kevin was so macho that he refused to wear much of the protection we were encouraged to don, so he winced at my kick.

Before I knew it, Kevin came at me with two quick punches, followed by a kick that didn't reach me. One of my advantages in this sport, I'd discovered, was the length of my legs. At times, people who had to spar with me would complain before the match even started. "It's not fair! Her legs are so long that I can't even get in there!" A quick and seasoned fighter had no problem figuring out how to get past my neophyte skills, but at this level, I could hold my own against the men. I responded to his effort with another satisfying "thwack" to his gut. I tried not to smile as I won another two points.

Kevin and I kept at it until we were told to stop and bow to each other, but not before he tried a few fancy spinning moves and landed some hard punches on me. I countered with my own set of aggressive moves, and at the end, it was energizing to meet Kevin's eyes, grasp our gloves, and bow in gratitude for a good match. I trotted back to the locker room, feeling like a million bucks.

It wasn't until I got into the car and was driving home that I realized I had crossed an invisible threshold during my match with Crazy Kevin. It couldn't have happened without actually putting myself into a fighting situation, though, something that had never before occurred in my adult life.

In this Hapkido studio, I was an adult woman who had been tutored in the art of fair fighting, learned to square off against a man without breaking gaze, and then end with ancient decorum and established rules. This hadn't been the case when I was a young girl; it was never a fair fight with my parents. Their blows had landed when I was defenseless and without warning. Endless hours of talking about this unequal dynamic in therapy had helped, but only up to a point, just as my father's indirect apology the day he died had only alleviated a tiny piece of that old pain.

Today, without even knowing what was happening or what was about to erupt in my psyche, I'd fought against an aggressive man and held my own, and had departed from our sparring match with dignity and strength. My Eureka moment in the car was that talking about this part of my life for years couldn't hold a candle to the emotional breakthrough I'd experienced while fighting a man within the confines of safe boundaries. I had no idea what the score of my match with Kevin was, but I knew I'd won an important victory in a routine class that had started inauspiciously.

I silently thanked Shep for yet another suggestion that had struck emotional gold. There was no way he could have anticipated that suggesting the martial arts for Samantha would open the door to giving me the tools required to heal one of the ugliest scars from my childhood. But it had, and I could see that more good lessons would emerge from this sport. In fact, if I could achieve the black belt level with my daughter, not only would I never see myself as a defenseless little girl again, I would have helped my daughter gain a certain cloak of confidence, like an invisible suit of armor, for the rest of her life.

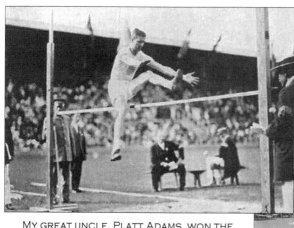

MY GREAT UNCLE, PLATT ADAMS, WON THE GOLD MEDAL AT THE 1912 OLYMPICS IN THE STANDING HIGH JUMP, WHICH SET THE BAR HIGH FOR ALL OF THE GOALS PURSUED IN OUR FAMILY.

HAYWOOD QUICKLY BECAME A NATIONALLY-RANKED SWIMMER BEFORE HE TURNED TEN, BUT ALL THREE CHILDREN LOVED THEIR SUMMER SWIM TEAM, MONTGOMERY SQUARE, SO THEY SPENT A LOT OF TIME IN BATHING SUITS WHEN THE WEATHER WAS WARM.

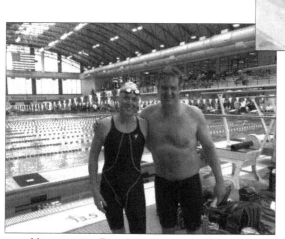

MY BROTHER, BILL ADAMS, DECIDED THAT IT HAD BEEN TOO LONG (35 YEARS) SINCE WE HAD SWUM IN THE SAME MEET, SO IN APRIL 2013 WE COMPETED TOGETHER AT THE COLONIES ZONES MEET AT GEORGE MASON UNIVERSITY, WHERE I WON SEVERAL EVENTS AND CAME CLOSE TO MANY OF MY HIGH SCHOOL BEST TIMES.

## CHAPTER TWENTY ONE
## WHAT'S NEXT?

One thing I had always longed for in my family was to be appreciated and "seen" for my uniqueness and individuality, but the qualities that differentiated me from others had always been criticized; conforming to a specific norm was what got rewarded. As a result, I'd never felt the freedom to do what I wanted, say what I wanted, write what I wanted, or even go where I wanted without being penalized. In fact, I'd never even been allowed to exist separately from my older sister Lizzie, and had always felt that my parents wanted a clone of her instead of the person I turned out to be. Just thirteen months apart, we'd been raised almost as twins, attending the same schools, doing the same sports, and even wearing the same clothes. Partly because of that, I wanted my children to grow up pursuing their own dreams, finding their own voices, and developing in ways that I might not agree with, but that allowed them to own the consequences of their choices. They might not look like the other perfect teen billboards who often emerged from this town—like me—but at least they'd be happier because they would have chosen their own paths.

So if my kids wanted to try something, I always found a way to get them there, but the rule was that if they started an activity or hobby that had a defined season, they had to finish it. No quitting.

By the age of eight, Haywood had tried basketball, lacrosse, wrestling, swimming, baseball, ice hockey, Cub Scouts, soccer, and piano lessons. To support him I'd volunteered in the Cub Scouts, built toy cars for the annual Pinewood Derby, made sure he had the right gear for every sport, and arranged and driven carpools that ate up my afternoons—if not entire days—during weekends, summers and school breaks. Some days I spent six full hours driving to and from various places, certain that my body was going to become indelibly imprinted on the driver's seat.

Haywood's entry into swimming had been inauspicious. At one of his Montessori teacher conferences, we had been told that he seemed to be uncoordinated and prone to getting injured, and his teacher thought we should consider getting him some swimming lessons to tame his energy and give him motor skill confidence. Since Haywood and I had both been competitive swimmers—I through my freshman year of college and Haywood until he was twelve—we liked the idea and immediately found him some group lessons at a local university.

I had decidedly mixed feelings about being around a pool, though, because I still associated the smell of chlorine with some of my worst years of bulimia. Just walking through the bathrooms that linked to indoor pool decks brought back waves of sadness. How many swim practices and meets had been compromised because I'd spent hours binging and purging that day or week, and I was too disoriented to focus on competing, or even too disgusted with my body to bear looking at myself in a bathing suit? Of all of the losses linked to my eating disorder, this was still one of the hardest to deal with. I had no idea what I might have achieved if I'd had a normal relationship with food, or confidence in my own abilities and body.

Despite my own bittersweet emotions, it was fun to watch Haywood take to the water with such joy, and to witness the peace and calm he felt after exhausting himself in the pool. His nature was so restless and driven that it was rare to see him tired, but as he progressed from lessons to local summer league meets to daily practices on year-round teams, it was obvious that swimming was the sport that gave him the most equilibrium and made him both happy and calm. It also brought him success. By the age of nine, he was winning a lot of breaststroke races, and at ten he was ranked 8th and 9th in the country in his two events, the 50- and 100-yard breaststroke.

I watched his progress with curiosity and fascination. I had been a breaststroker, as had my husband. This stroke appeared to be an inborn talent, one that was hard to teach to someone who wasn't naturally inclined. Breaststroke requires a certain type of rhythm that lets the body surge forward while also briefly pausing with every kick, making it one of the most exhausting—and slowest—events to swim. The stroke also favors people who walk like a duck because of the frog-like kick required for propulsion. The other three strokes—freestyle, backstroke and butterfly—lean more heavily on sheer power, particularly in the shorter races.

Seeing Haywood excel, and begin to travel around the country breaking records, changed our family in fundamental ways. Swimming is one of the few sports you need to commit to on a daily basis, often with two-a-day workouts starting at a young age, with rare time off lest you lose the "feel" of the water. Although we held out as long as possible, Haywood had to gradually taper off his participation in anything that conflicted with swim practice, which meant that I found myself driving to multiple swim practices for different swim teams on a regular basis, often dragging Bayard and Samantha along. Some weekends featured all-day swim meets, many with competitions that had trial heats in the mornings with finals at night.

Haywood had clearly found the thing that brought him both satisfaction and success. Samantha was thriving in the martial arts, and both of them were excellent students. Despite the time our family had to devote to swimming, Samantha continued to take piano lessons and be a Girl Scout, so she never felt that she wasn't getting enough attention or had to make onerous sacrifices for her brother. She also enjoyed competing on our summer league swim teams because she developed an entirely different set of friends there than those from school.

When it came to Bayard, however, a whole new set of challenges were already apparent at a very young age—challenges that would require a very different set of mothering skills and patience that I wasn't sure I possessed. To put it bluntly, Bayard was not a happy child. Starting with the anxious gaze he'd fixed on me at the moment of his birth, it was hard to find anything that made him content for very long. All of our family pictures during this period feature two smiling children and one scared little boy, warily taking it all in. The first time I saw a genuine smile on his face, I noticed that he had grown two bottom teeth without my even registering that milestone because it was so rare that he gave me a joyful, open-mouthed grin.

By the time Bayard was one, though, he discovered something that seemed to give him peace, something that allowed him to lose track of time without throwing a tantrum or crying in abject sadness. I was making dinner one night when I found out what it was.

It was early 1996, and I was cooking spaghetti and garlic bread. Despite my well-known sub-par cooking skills, there are a few things I can make that everyone will eat, and this was one of those meals. I had just dumped the spaghetti in the boiling water while my nine-month-old toddler sat behind me on the kitchen floor, playing with the colorful plastic magnetic letters on the refrigerator door.

Suddenly he erupted with an utterance. "A!" he called out happily.

I turned around to see a grinning little boy, triumphantly reaching out towards me with a purple letter A in his chubby fingers. I walked over to the refrigerator and knelt down to his level.

"That's right Bayard," I said with some surprise. "It's an A." I took the letter out of his hand and put it back on the refrigerator and selected a red letter "I." "What's this?" I held it up in front of him.

"I," he replied without hesitation. Then he picked another letter and cried out excitedly, "B!" and handed me a blue lower-case B. This went on for some time as Bayard accurately named every letter either one of us selected.

I went back to making dinner but couldn't stop thinking about what had just happened. Had Haywood and Samantha recognized letters before they could articulate sentences, too? Haywood had known car company insignias and was able to solve puzzles quickly, but knowing letters didn't resonate with me. Samantha had been a blast of non-stop talking and singing, sometimes in endless stuttering loops, but letters didn't come to mind as part of her development, either. I decided to ask Haywood that night what he thought about what I'd witnessed.

"Have you ever noticed that Bayard knows the letters of the alphabet? He recognized every letter on the refrigerator and was accurate every time he handed me one or I picked one and showed it to him. Did Haywood and Samantha do that? I honestly can't remember."

The truth was that I was not only unable to remember my other two children's childhoods in detail at this point, I was so exhausted that I could barely think straight at times. Samantha had only started to sleep through the night when Bayard was born, which had led to many disrupted nights while I was pregnant, and had probably contributed to my being sick at the time of his birth. Now I was trying to make an anxious baby happy while running the other two around all day, and it was taking a toll on my own wellbeing and energy level, not to mention my ability to feel like I had a working brain.

On the opposite end of the spectrum, my husband actually looked younger and fresher to me at 35 and had even been asked for identification recently when he tried to buy beer. It was obvious that having a job he loved and being able to travel whenever he needed to without giving the childcare situation a second thought, was good for him. As a result, he rarely ran out of steam or was anything other than good-natured.

I occasionally envied my husband's life and wished I had figured out a better way to balance motherhood with my desire to do my own things. But since nothing really felt professionally compelling enough to turn my children over to nannies and babysitters, I found myself putting down deeper and deeper roots, staying home and gradually becoming the equivalent of a full-time driver, housekeeper, cook and babysitter.

As we discussed Bayard's predilection for letters that night, Haywood couldn't recall our other children having similar aptitudes, but we agreed that the hours of staring at "Sesame Street" had probably given Bayard a head start on learning the alphabet that perhaps the others hadn't had. On multiple occasions we had both watched him planted in front of the show with an unblinking stare, intently absorbing everything he saw on the screen. Maybe he was watching too much television, I chided myself. Was I parking Bayard in front of shows to buy myself a few minutes here and there to take a shower or do something of my own? I'd have to be careful of that.

It turned out that the episode with letters was just the beginning of some other eyebrow-raising events. One day when Bayard was about 18 months old, I walked into his room where he was perched on a chair playing a computer game called "Reader Rabbit" that challenged players to identify words that matched clues on the screen. Standing silently behind him, I watched Bayard effortlessly match every word with every clue. How could he do that? Had he memorized the screen and all of the cues by watching his brother and sister play?

I walked over to the computer and put Bayard on my lap.

"Can I play with you for a few minutes?" I asked. "This looks like fun and I haven't done this with you in a while." I maneuvered the mouse to take me to a more difficult part of the game with a more complicated set of word challenges.

"I do it," he said angrily, pushing my hand off the mouse and moving it quickly to the right answer. He did this several more times, never making an error. I sat there astonished. I knew Bayard recognized letters, but was my child now reading words and understanding clues that were tailored to a second grade audience? It was certainly puzzling, but if it kept him happy, I wasn't going to mess with the pleasure he appeared to be getting.

One day I left a credit card on the dining room table and Bayard walked over to the table, picked it up, and carried it into the kitchen to me.

"US Air" he said happily. I looked down at the card, and it saw that it was a USAir Visa card, but there was no image of an airplane on the card that might have cued him in to name an airline company. How had he figured that one out? Another time he walked past a black armchair featuring a decal from our college. "Harvard," he said, as sauntered past, glancing at the chair.

Unsure of exactly what he was doing or what it meant, I took him to a homeopathic doctor who combined Western medical training with an alternative approach to health. Although I had both feet firmly in the camp of using a traditional pediatrician most of the time, I occasionally supplemented my children's care with the gentle impact of the homeopathic remedies and I trusted this doctor's judgment on things that fell outside the normal spectrum of health questions. I wanted his perspective before I went any further.

"Dr. Aurigemma," I said one morning. "I think my son is reading, but I can't be completely sure if he has just memorized letters and words because he's heard people say what they are, and he's parroting it back, or if he really understands what he's seeing. I'm not even sure if he has memorized my handwriting and can associate the words I write with the sounds he's heard that go along with them. Would you mind putting these words in your own handwriting to see if he can read them off a piece of paper? It just all seems a little bit strange to me."

Dr. Aurigemma was a funky guy, with a friendly Brooklyn accent and an open-minded approach, but he still looked a little skeptical as I slid a piece of paper across his desk. I'd written words like "Harvard," "USAir," "Washington," and "Hi." All told it was about twenty words that Bayard had recognized at some point. I threw in a few challenge words that I didn't think he'd ever seen before, just as a test.

The doctor frowned slightly, then copied the words in a mixture of block letters and upper-case and lower-case letters. He pushed it back to me and I held it up in front of Bayard, who sat on my lap holding his bottle of juice. "Can you tell me what this says?" I asked.

Without missing a beat, Bayard rattled off the words. Dr. Aurigemma sat behind his desk, momentarily speechless. "I don't think I've ever seen anything like that," he finally offered.

He asked me a few more questions to try to understand why I might have a toddler who was reading with relative ease and proficiency despite not having parents who had ever tried to force that skill. He also wanted to know more about what kinds of things and situations made him unhappy.

Although I'd talked to Shep about Bayard, and he'd suggested that I visit a child psychologist for some testing, I'd resisted it. I wasn't sure I wanted to start down a road of giving my child labels before the age of two, but I was definitely concerned that with the exception of words and atlases, there wasn't much that made Bayard happy.

I exhaled and began to talk. "He won't wear shoes because he says shoes shouldn't touch the ground and ever get dirty. If I don't give in to some of his quirks, like not wearing shoes from time to time, I can't get through the day."

"What else does he do that concerns you?"

"He won't wear shirts or clothing unless they have words on them. He calls things by the name he sees on the product—like London Fog for a coat, Evenflo for a bottle, or Rubbermaid for a cup—and gets angry if we don't call it by the same name that he uses. He screams for hours if we try to leave him with sitters, because they don't understand him. One night we got a call from a neighborhood girl who was practically in tears because Bayard wanted a certain stuffed animal to go to bed with, and when she tried to get him to describe it, he kept screaming that it was a stuffed animal that had a "Y" for a mouth."

I went on. "He carries books and atlases around with him, and he likes facts, but if something isn't a fact, like during Halloween when people are trick-or-treating and dressed differently, he freaks out and hides. I'm worried that he'll never really be able to socialize with anyone unless I get some comprehension of what is going on his brain. I don't understand my own child, and because of that, I feel like I can't be a good parent to him. I feel overwhelmed by how different he is from my other two."

Dr. Aurigemma tapped his pencil on his desk. He thought for a moment. Then he asked if I was familiar with a man in Bethesda who had a worldwide reputation for manipulating energy to heal people. "I think you should see Mietek Wirkus," he said. "He's been studied by scientists and there have been documentaries done about him, and pictures taken of his hands with special types of Kirlian photography. He lectures around the world and does private readings because of the impact he has on people when he focuses his energy on them. Why don't we start with something that can't do any harm, just to see what he says and what impact he has on Bayard?"

There was a famous energy healer in Bethesda who had magical hands? This was a new piece of information to me. I'd been born and raised here, and I'd never heard of such a thing, but if this well-trained doctor sitting in front of me thought he might help Bayard, I was going to try. My openness to "woo woo" philosophies had begun during my early years of recovery in Baltimore, where I'd explored as many avenues as possible that might assist in my healing. At that time, I'd looked into New Age thinking, meditation, past life therapy and even astrology. I felt that if anything could help me recover from my eating disorder and get stronger without doing harm, who was I to judge it? So if something unusual could cut into my son's anxiety now and improve the quality of his life, would it be responsible for me to simply ignore it because it was unconventional?

Within a week I was standing in the office of Mietek Wirkus, who charged a pittance to meet individuals, read their energies, and then do some breathing while he moved his hands carefully up and down their body to balance their energies, hovering about a foot away, his eyes never leaving the spot he was focusing on. His English was rudimentary, so the office was overseen by his wife and some other assistants who were more fluent in the language, but it didn't seem necessary to exchange words with him, anyway. He just smiled a hello and then assumed a relaxed stance, one foot in front of the other, as he went to work.

Bayard was uncharacteristically accepting of this man whom he'd never met. As I cradled my young son in my arms I gazed around the office to try to get more insight into Mietek. It was small and unpretentious, without any obvious New Age symbols, but something odd caught my attention that I'd never seen before. A common houseplant sat on a desk, but it had grown up and out of the pot, and now stretched up the side wall, where a grate had clearly been installed for the plant to grab onto. From there, the plant crawled all the way up the wall and bent its way onto the ceiling, stopping after a few feet. It was a vibrant, healthy green, but where did you get a plant like this? I couldn't help asking, hoping he would understand my question.

"What kind of plant is this?" I gestured to the pot.

Mietek smiled and answered. "A sick plant. I wanted to…" he searched for the right words, "make it better. The energy in here is good. The plant is happy. You can see." He waved his hand up at the ceiling and then went back to work, his hands now close to Bayard's cap of curly blond hair.

Wow. Could it be that Mietek's energy was so strong, and so good, that a dying plant could literally explode with life and grow into gargantuan proportions? I didn't know what to think, but if he had that type of life-giving power, I hoped he could help Bayard be a little happier, too.

After ten minutes, Mietek stepped away from Bayard, hands dropping to his side to indicate he was finished. He gestured to Bayard. "Brain is on fire. He can't turn it off. It is making him sad. I think I quieted it down a little bit, though. Very hot when I started." His hands pantomimed being burned.

Although I had no context for this input, it made sense that my son's brain was on fire. That's what it felt like to me—it seemed like Bayard could never stop thinking long enough to just be a little boy and find joy in stupid things, like rolling a plastic truck on the ground or playing with Legos. Maybe the wires in his brain were crossed in such a way that he needed help untangling them long enough to rest his thinking, and if this helped, who was I to criticize it?

I slung my somnolent child slung over my shoulder and walked to my car, where I strapped Bayard into his child seat. He was asleep even before we pulled out of the parking spot. I put him into bed when I got home; he looked as if he'd been knocked out. In fact, I even felt a bit dreamy and calmer myself. What was this effect Mietek had had on us?

More than 24 hours later Bayard woke up, as if emerging from a drugged sleep. Although I couldn't prove that anything had occurred during that visit, it appeared to me that Mietek had intervened to give Bayard a small respite from the intensity of his brain. Perhaps he shifted things around so that the learning or processing could occur in a different way.

Regardless, I felt like I had confirmation from a stranger that something very intense was happening in my little boy's head.

The rest of 1996 and into 1997 were eye-opening because the pace of Bayard's development accelerated. Friends who dropped by with their children for play dates began to witness his precocious reading if he felt comfortable enough to do it in front of them. More than once my friends said, "You ought to get that kid onto Letterman!" If Bayard didn't know our visitor extremely well, he would shut down and bury his head in my shoulder, often begging to be taken from the room.

If we went out to a new place and Bayard got scared, he would only calm down if he identified letters around him that he could talk about. Once, cowering in his familiar place in my arms, head down and his eyes on the ground, I heard a happy exclamation.

"It's a J!" he screamed in delight, pointing at the floor. I looked down and stared at the rubber shapes that stretched across the floor of the vast auditorium. I realized that the entire area was, indeed, a set of interlocking J's, all jumbled up in such a way that I never would have spotted myself, but it was all Bayard saw.

When Haywood took Bayard to the National Zoo, where the famous Chinese pandas are on display and every exotic beast known to man is housed, Bayard never seemed to see the animals. I found this out when he came home and I tried to talk to him about his experience.

"How was the zoo? What did you see? Did you have fun?"

On one occasion, Bayard informed me that he had seen the words "Push" and "Thank You" on the doors and signs he had encountered. Another time he went into the Amazonia exhibit and noticed that an entire wall of the building had a projected visual of its nine South American countries, and it wasn't long before he had found the computer that controlled the wall and was in charge. Haywood recounted to me that while dozens of other children oohed and aahed about the jaguars and anaconda snakes, my son had busily clicked through the pictures and facts of the various countries that comprised Amazonia, keeping the wall display in motion as he absorbed new nuggets of knowledge.

The most unforgettable moment, though, was the afternoon I pulled up in front of a 7-11 convenience store in my minivan, my almost five year-old daughter at my side and Bayard strapped into his car seat right behind me.

Samantha, who was beginning to expand her vocabulary as her reading progressed, looked at the banner hanging along the front of the store.

"Mommy, what's a mug?"

Before I had a moment to turn the key in the ignition to off, or answer her, we heard Bayard's voice echo through the car.

"It's for fresh hot coffee," he said.

I glanced up at the banner that read, "Cool new mug for fresh hot coffee," and my mouth dropped open. I turned around to stare incredulously at Bayard, and the first thing I noticed was his plastic diaper, which seemed incongruous in light of what had just happened. In the blink of an eye, my two-year-old son had heard his older sister's question, read the banner, digested the information, and spat out an answer.

This was a first for me. Mietek was right—my son's brain was on fire and nothing seemed to be able to slow it down. How was I going to keep up with him and give him the right parenting he needed? This was a "gift" he'd been born with, but like a rose has thorns, it was clearly accompanied by sadness when there weren't enough words or letters to satisfy his brain.

We decided that the first step was to get him into the Montessori School that had been so wonderful for Haywood and Samantha. Although he was a little young even by their liberal standards, they agreed to have him come for two hours every morning, with a pick-up just before lunch. I wanted to get their perspective on Bayard's academic readiness without my input, so I simply said that Bayard was prepared to meet some new children and socialize, and left out everything else.

Despite his unease with new people and situations, Bayard had been in the car every day that I had dropped off and picked up his brother and sister, so the faces that came to the car at the beginning and end of every

196

school day were familiar to him, and therefore not threatening. He was also especially close to his siblings, so walking into school with his sister, and even into the same classroom, wasn't a problem. I drove away, hoping that the morning would be a success.

Within an hour, the phone rang. "Caroline, this is Joan Smith." Joan was the unflappable, no-nonsense teacher who headed up the classroom where Bayard and Samantha were placed. I prayed that this wasn't a call that Bayard couldn't stay.

"Did you know that Bayard can read?"

I burst out with relief and laughter. "Yes, but I wanted you to see it for yourself. Sometimes he hides it if he's in a new or uncomfortable setting with people he doesn't know. I wasn't sure what was going to happen today."

"Well, it was hard to hide it when he met the aide in his classroom," Joan chuckled. "He pointed right at her breasts and said, 'Abercrombie and Fitch.' Later we found him near the air conditioner, reading the instructions on the outside. How long has this been going on?"

I explained what we'd observed, starting at nine months, along with my own concerns about how words were the only things that Bayard truly seemed to love. She promised to keep an eye on him and give me feedback about how he was fitting into the classroom, although she assured me that he'd have some six-year-olds to read with, so he wouldn't feel so alone. Later I learned that everyone in his class had been given atlases, too, so that when Bayard wanted to talk about and look at countries, rivers, mountains and other geographical facts, he would have company.

A few months later, I heard a knock in the early afternoon on the front door. I opened it to see Joan Smith standing there, holding a sheaf of papers. She didn't look upset, so it couldn't be bad, but I'd never had a teacher visit my house, so I was concerned.

"I don't want to interrupt anything," she said, holding out the papers in her hand, "but I think you need to read this. It might be the key to understanding Bayard." She quickly departed, leaving me with a surprising set of facts about a learning disability I'd never heard of: hyperlexia.

I found a chair in the kitchen and slowly took in everything she'd given me. Joan had copied printouts from a wide variety of medical and psychological websites that seemed to describe my child to a "T," but with some alarming side-effects that could accompany this diagnosis.

Hyperlexia was the opposite of dyslexia, it explained, with the primary feature being a precocious ability to read before the age of two, usually with an uncontrollable compulsion that the child can't regulate. These children were gifted, but anxious, because they could take in vast amounts of adult information, but they couldn't process it or put into a normal emotional framework or context because they were so young.

I immediately thought of a recent experience where Bayard had been walking through the kitchen, his blue baby blanket around his neck. He'd looked up at the television and asked, "What is 'The Crisis in Kosovo'?" It was obvious if there were words anywhere in Bayard's vicinity, he didn't have the ability to choose NOT to read them; he HAD to read them. Trying to answer upsetting questions in childish terms undid him even more because he frequently had taken in more data than we knew, and if our explanations didn't match the facts in his head, he'd get troubled. I'd started to hide the newspapers from Bayard and keep the news off as much as possible because so much of what was in the media was negative and frightening. Was hyperlexia why Bayard had so much anxiety all the time? Just how early had he started to absorb things I didn't even know about?

I kept reading. Hyperlexic children not only showed an early fascination with letters and numbers, they didn't like anything that wasn't factual and had difficulty with abstract concepts. A bell went off in my head. This explained why Bayard read *National Geographic* magazines and atlases in every free minute—they were factual. We'd even invested in a 9-foot by 15-foot map of the world and put it on one entire wall of his room because looking at maps transfixed and soothed him.

Halloween was *not* factual, so Bayard's brain didn't have a place to park the concept that people would dress as something they are not. In fact, his first experience with the Montessori school on a Halloween had started with Joan coming to the car dressed as a black cat, and it had sent Bayard into paroxysms of misery. "Nobody is who they are supposed to be!" he wailed, as I took him back home to sit out the fun holiday with me.

The inability to cope with abstract ideas, and to jump to erroneous conclusions about commonplace events, was also a feature of their thinking. I understood that, too, because it had manifested itself already. For example, Bayard had seen his brother open a wallet in the kitchen one afternoon, and he'd run out of the room, wailing. When I caught up with him he explained in gasping sobs that he didn't have a wallet yet, and that not having a wallet meant that he had no money, and no money and no wallet meant he'd grow up to be a poor adult. Following his thinking as it leapt around was a perplexing challenge that was hard to keep up with—and harder still to know how to respond to it.

Hyperlexic children also have extreme sensitivity to touch, which now explained why he couldn't wear shoes, and would scream if his shirt had something as insignificant as a drop of water on it. His whole sensory process was on fire and he had no control over it, just like his brain, and in many ways he was a helpless victim of something he seemed to have been born with. Again, I thought about Mietek describing Bayard's brain as a raging forest fire. Although he hadn't had a formal diagnosis for Bayard in western medical terms, he'd hit the nail on the burning head.

The most troubling parts of the hyperlexia definitions stated that some children—because the disorder was on a spectrum with a number of autism characteristics that may or may not be present—would never be able to be mainstreamed into a formal school setting, and that socializing with children who didn't see the world in the same way might be too hard for them.

Tears filled my eyes. Was this going to be Bayard's fate? I knew that my own life had ground to a halt as I'd tried to integrate him into our family while trying to be patient and understanding of his differences, but this was a whole new area of parenting that was uncharted territory. Was he going to require homeschooling? I had already decided that going back to any type of work was not going to happen for me soon because I didn't know anyone besides me and Haywood—and occasionally his siblings—who could calm Bayard down when necessary. Babysitters, *au pairs* and nannies had not worked out for a variety of reasons, and even my brother and sister-in-law felt overwhelmed when I left him with them for brief periods.

"Don't mention global warning or tornados," I cautioned my sister-in-law when she came by to help one afternoon. Although taken aback, she'd tried to keep conversations at a pre-school level. Any random mention of something Bayard had read about that had potentially bad outcomes could cause hysteria that went on and on, and very few people had the willingness to hang in there with him until it ended.

One fresh example of why I couldn't turn Bayard over to a random caregiver came to mind. On weekends, many of the realty companies have open houses to show their properties, and one of the biggest realtors is called "W.C. & A.N. Miller," or "Miller" for short. I'd been doing some type of errand with Bayard and the other two kids in the car when Bayard had suddenly become very upset.

"Miller Open House!" he screamed unhappily. "Why is our house open? These are not all of our houses! They are not Miller houses!"

Suddenly, it seemed like the world was a sea of red and white signs that all proclaimed that there were Miller Open Houses on every street, and Bayard didn't have any idea how to conceptualize and accept that they were not about *our* house.

I snapped in exasperation, begging Bayard to stop crying and to just "be normal." I felt bad the moment I said it, but my mothering skills were fraying in the face of these unpredictable onslaughts. I'd had to abort countless activities when Bayard had a meltdown that no one else could have possibly understood. I felt like I was on my last nerve and that my life had telescoped down to trying to stay one step ahead of Bayard's thinking and anxieties so that we could have relative calm in the house.

On other occasions, we'd be on the highway, where there were announcements of "local" lanes, and Bayard would insist that we move into the "local" lanes because he liked the word "local" better than "express." He also developed an affinity for signs that read "bumps ahead," but none of us understood why. Fortunately, on summer days when I picked Haywood and Samantha up from their camps, and Bayard got into a snit, they'd tolerantly let me drive around until I found enough "bumps ahead" signs to soothe Bayard back into complacency. They were already developing protectiveness for their brother, who was clearly not a run-of-the-mill child, and they wanted him to be happy, too.

I shuffled through the papers Joan had left with me. Hyperlexia was clearly what we were dealing with, but I wasn't sure where Bayard fell on the spectrum. Finding that out, and then constructing an environment of supports and guidance so that he had a fighting chance to accept himself in all of his uniqueness, had to be my top priority. My own life, whatever that was going to be, would have to wait.

I suddenly remembered the way I'd felt when I found out that my parents had received my ADHD diagnosis as a young child, but had ignored it and let the situation advance to the point where I settled into self-destructive behaviors like bulimia because it had calmed me down when I couldn't turn off my own energies and run-on thinking. I had been outside the norm, too, but my parents hadn't had the desire or energy to address my needs with either compassion or professional advice. Instead, they'd treated me like a mistake, trying to get rid of me as often and as quickly as possible.

I understood how they felt, but I wasn't going to abandon Bayard. I didn't know how this was going to turn out, or even how I would cope with whatever surprises lay ahead, but this much was clear: if I didn't create the environment Bayard required to thrive and feel loved, no one else was going to do it.

## CHAPTER TWENTY TWO
## HAVING IT ALL?

When Bayard was a baby, we sat for a family portrait at the neighborhood park in the matching pale outfits photographers favor. As we sat down on a blanket, the sun dappling through the branches of the towering trees, our faces softened with warm light, the photographer muttered under his breath, "This is always the hardest spacing of children to photograph... this isn't going to be fun."

As he coached us through poses and smiles, together and separately, it became obvious what he was talking about. Haywood was doing his usual hyperactive routine, barely sitting still and begging to run off and play on the swings every few minutes. Whenever he was coaxed into compliance, either Bayard or Samantha needed attention or wanted to crawl away. We eventually got our family picture and Christmas card shot, but the age and energy mismatches definitely made it an exhausting afternoon, which mirrored many of the frustrations I found myself living with as they got older and the days became more complex.

I often thought about the photographer's observation as parenting became my full-time gig, while my professional identity became a distant, foggy memory. With gaps of two to three years between each child, it was unusual to have any of them at the same developmental level at any one time, so they couldn't be parked together in similar activities that gave me a small break to do my own thing for long. For example, when Haywood was able to swim, Samantha was in the early stages of learning to float and couldn't be left alone in the shallow end of the pool, while Bayard wasn't even able to leave the confines of the baby pool.

Bayard continued to require extra attention, but the Montessori school became his bright spot because of the innovative teaching methods that allowed him to progress at a rate that was appropriate for him. As time went on, he developed friendships with boys and girls who understood that he saw the world differently than they did, but they still liked him and wanted to play with him.

Despite our early concerns about hyperlexia, Bayard never completely met all of the criteria, including the ones that would have prevented him from bonding with others. He landed somewhere in the middle of the spectrum, demonstrating many of its notable features, but not the extremes such as being unable to make eye contact, or not having the skills to communicate effectively enough to make friends. It also helped us tremendously when Bayard began to work with a skillful child psychiatrist who was able to help him frame his thoughts and fears so that he wouldn't come to conclusions that didn't serve him well.

Some motherhood days were harder than others for me. I often went to the local park with the children on nice days, pushing my orange double jog stroller, trying to get into the ethos of just hanging out and killing time. For many, this was a breeze, but with my ADHD, activities like this often moved too slowly and I felt like my time there was akin to watching grass grow.

One desultory day, I took my children to the park where I stood surrounded by multiple foreign nannies, and didn't see a single friendly mom face I knew. I watched the kids happily running around, but before long, impatience had sunk in and I couldn't pretend that the park was the desirable option I wanted that afternoon. Did other mommies hate the park? Was there something wrong with me? Is that why so many moms had full-time nannies, whether they worked outside the home or not... because it was easier to pay someone to do things like this?

I knew I wasn't alone in my growing discontent of feeling underemployed and wondering where my life was heading if I continued to stay home and on this treadmill indefinitely. The *Washington Post* frequently wrote articles about how the town was filled with women like me who currently served as overqualified class mothers instead of professional go-getters, and who were now consumed by volunteer jobs at their children's schools instead of filing legal briefs or running political campaigns.

Every August I received a daunting packet of positions from the public schools requesting that we fill jobs ranging from Carnival co-chairs to field trip monitors. I knew lots of mothers who had gotten sucked into dozens of positions that seemed to piggyback on each other, and they were never able to extricate themselves from the frequent pleas to take on a few more tasks, leading to year after year of hundreds of hours of unpaid work. I dipped my toe into these waters a few times, but one incident underscored some of the frustrations that were rising within me.

My job as chair of the Silent Auction one spring was to gather as many donated services from the surrounding areas as I could to raise money to supplement the school's operating expenses. I decided to only approach places that I knew school parents frequently patronized, so one morning I went to a local coffee bar where I often stopped after finishing the morning carpool runs and socialized with other school moms.

I smiled as I walked into the bar. "I'd like to get my normal drink," I said to the familiar face behind the cash register, "but could I also ask the store to make a donation to our school's Silent Auction? Maybe ten free coffee drinks or something like that?" I smiled in certainty that this wouldn't be too much to ask for; I assumed they'd probably throw in a few bags of coffee, too.

"Just a moment. Let me go ask the store owner if that's okay." He disappeared into the back office.

A few moments later a small older woman with a face like a thundercloud emerged. "Can I help you?" she asked imperiously, looking me up and down.

Suddenly I felt like I'd done something wrong, and wasn't sure how to proceed. "Um, our school just up the street is having a Silent Auction and…" I could already tell that this conversation was going south, but I forged ahead. "Since so many of the parents, like me, come here all the time for coffee and other things, I thought you might be willing to support us with something like a gift card..."

The woman cut me off dismissively. "I'll give you a gift basket, but that's all," she answered, turning away to end the conversation. But she wasn't done with me. As she was about to re-enter the office she turned and looked at me. "Do you work?"

I wanted to tell her that I worked all the time, and that there wasn't a moment when I wasn't on call, or doing something for my husband and children. I wanted to tell her that I cooked, drove, scrubbed floors, did the laundry, cut the grass, painted, sewed and did just about every job around the house that needed to be done, and that I was exhausted most of the time. I also wanted to tell her that what I was doing was far harder than anything I'd ever done in an office where I got paid. In fact, I often thought that my days would be a lot more fun and rewarding if I got dressed up, looked nice, and left my house for other people to run while I pursued my own goals.

I shook my head.

"Lady, the next time you ask someone for something, make sure you get paid for it. It will feel a lot better." With her *coup de grace*, she exited the room.

I felt humiliated. All I'd done was ask for a small donation for a cause I believed in, and she'd made me feel inferior because I wasn't getting paid to do it. I put my coffee back on the counter and glanced at the cashier, who looked completely abashed by what he had just witnessed. "I'm sorry," he mumbled. "She can be like that."

＊ ＊ ＊ ＊ ＊ ＊ ＊ ＊ ＊

MY INTERACTION WITH the coffee shop owner crystallized my discontent. I lived in an uncomfortable netherworld of knowing I was doing something important by being home with my children, but I also longed to do more with my brain... and I missed getting paid for producing something that was

205

valuable to others. I also wanted my children to see that I was capable of doing something other than the household duties they saw me performing. Samantha, at least, understood that I had written some books because she'd asked why there were framed pictures of me on magazine covers around the house. I'd also spoken periodically at the elementary school when different professions were showcased, so on some level all three kids knew that I'd achieved prominence with what I'd done before they were born.

Samantha surprised me one morning when she came down dressed for school in my clothes. She'd found a sleeveless blue shirt that I often wore, and had paired it with my favorite distinctive wrap-around skirt featuring boats going around the hem in vibrant blues. She'd wrapped the skirt twice around her small waist, and was even wearing my shoes.

She smiled broadly when she saw my surprise. "What are you doing, Sam?" I asked. "Why are you in my clothes?" I put my hands on my hips and looked at her. "And my espadrilles?" She was already taller than all of her peers, but with my espadrilles she was going to be taller than her teacher.

"Today is 'Dress As Your Hero Day'" she explained. "I'm dressing like you because I want to grow up and write books like you!"

While I was touched, it was also poignant to hear her say that she wanted to do what I used to do, but not what I was doing now.

"That's sweet honey," I said. "Why do you want to write books?"

"Because everyone says you helped so many people with what you've written," she said. "I'd like to help people, too."

Samantha gradually became more aware of what I had written about because I began to share more details about my past life with bulimia, and how I'd gotten better. She asked lots of questions about how my eating disorder had started and what people had said about my body that had been so hard to cope with. She talked about girls in her class who said that they were fat and needed to diet, and also told me that a lot of her friends said that their mothers hated their bodies and were always dieting, too. Once a friend of hers had sat in my kitchen eating an after-school snack, and I'd eaten half a grilled cheese sandwich along with them. The girl had asked in surprise if

I usually ate during the day because her mom took diet pills in the morning so she wouldn't eat during the day.

I decided to bring Samantha in on more of the details of what my eating disorder actually meant beyond issues around food. So I took her to my annual Ob/Gyn appointment and specifically asked for a bone density scan so that I could explain what it meant to Samantha, and why it mattered to people like me.

She stood next to me as my wrist was scanned with a Dexa machine, and during the painless twenty-minute exam, I explained why I wanted her to see it.

"My eating disorder caused a lot of damage to my body, and some of the damage was invisible. People who did what I did could hurt their bones and make it easier for them to break, but still look normal on the outside," I said. "That's why you can't always know if someone has an eating disorder just by looking at them."

Samantha took it all in, asking "Are you okay now?"

The aide answered for her. "Your mom's bones are perfect."

I nodded. "Even if you do damage to your body, if you start to get better, a lot of things can be turned around, " I explained. "I've been recovering for a long time now, and because of that, my body has been able to heal." That satisfied her, but it also whetted her appetite for more.

"Can I read your book, mom?" When she was in seventh grade, she was able to understand more of the nuances of what I'd gone through, and after talking to Haywood, we agreed that she was old enough to learn about some of the more unsavory aspects of my life, particularly because I would be right there to answer her questions.

Samantha disappeared into her room one Sunday morning, and only came out after she'd finished the entire book many hours later. I looked at her face expectantly.

"What did you think?" I held my breath, wondering what she'd thought about mom smoking marijuana, which actually concerned me more than the binging scenes I'd revealed.

"I learned a lot," she said.

"Like what?"

"Dad wanted to walk fast out of the Cathedral when you got married," she said. "Also, you threw up a lot at Harvard, but people helped you get better through that group you joined later. Do you still talk to them?"

That was all she learned? Where was the horror and shock about the gory details?

"So the book didn't scare you?"

"No, why would it?"

"Well, there was a lot of stuff in there that I hadn't told you before, and I thought it might be hard for you to read."

"No, not really," she said matter-of-factly. "I'm glad I read it because I understand more of what you went through, but you've never hidden it from me, either, or pretended you were perfect when you were younger. I think I'd be more shocked if you'd never said anything about bulimia and I suddenly found out now." She frowned as she thought of an analogy that would make sense. "It would be like suddenly finding out you were adopted at my age."

She had just taught me something important. Because there had been no blueprint for much of my recovery, and then for how to raise children while staying in recovery, I'd been groping my way through it for years, hoping I was handling all of the different situations well, doing as much as possible in my power to avoid some of the pitfalls I'd had.

Samantha had just let me know that my nonchalant attitude about my bulimic history, and the fact that I'd never hidden it, but certainly hadn't forced details on her unless she asked, had been the right approach for her. She had knowledge of something that was already impacting girls her age, and that was undoubtedly still hurting some of her friends' mothers, but she also had the benefit of knowing that people got better.

Within a few months of Samantha's reading my book, I had an opportunity to show her another way to identify invisible damage from my past and heal it. We were in downtown Bethany on a hot summer day in the week before school started, and we passed a boutique with a huge sign: "50% off on all bathing suits." I suddenly remembered one of my bucket list items. I grabbed her hand and said, "Come on... let's go buy a bikini."

I was forty years old and I'd still never worn a bikini. This was my chance to take a stand against my old demons that had once told me that bikinis were only for drop-dead gorgeous women with great bodies. Just as I'd once thought hot food was taboo, and eating a piece of quiche would send me back into bulimia, this was my chance to tell my subconscious that I could wear a bikini and it wasn't restricted to some version of a pretty woman that I couldn't be.

We headed to the back of the store where the on-sale bathing suits hung. Most of them looked silly to me, with gold hardware, fringes and neon colors. There's no way I'd wear any of them in public. I quickly flipped through them, and then my eyes lit upon a simple black suit. It wasn't frivolous or too revealing, and black signified sophistication to me. Wearing a black bikini would mean that I'd really changed some important channels in my brain about who I was.

As I tried on and paid for the bathing suit, I explained to Samantha why it was so important to me that I buy it. She tried to understand my point as I told her that I'd always "hidden" myself in one-piece Speedo racing suits. Even though they were skintight, they still camouflaged my fear of looking flawed. Because Samantha had grown up being comfortable slipping from her swim team bathing suit into a bikini when she was with her friends, she didn't really understand what the big deal was.

Later that week, on the beach, in as unpopulated an area as possible, I did the "big reveal" of the bikini. My first reaction was that I'd never had any air on my stomach outside the privacy of my own home, and it made me feel vulnerable and strange to feel it. But I hung in there for the afternoon, gradually adapting to a world I'd never permitted myself to enter, wondering how I'd ever let something as inconsequential as wearing a bikini become such a limiting fear.

* * * * * * * *

While working with Kathleen I'd successfully wrestled through my working mom dilemmas—first to write a book when Haywood was a baby, and then later to briefly work part-time when Samantha was young, while also writing three more books (one was ghostwritten for someone else and I couldn't disclose who it was) right up until the day I had Bayard. Maybe book-writing was all I could do with small kids, I'd reasoned, so I'd sent my agent some chapters of a novel I'd written. I was crushed when she not only told me she didn't like my ideas, she but she also said she couldn't represent me any longer. She recommended me to two other agents, but neither of them thought I was worthy of being represented either, so I'd regretfully concluded that my writing days were over.

It was difficult for me to imagine what I could do. Without an agent, it would be nearly impossible to get published again. I was a middle-aged professional failure, I began to worry. I wasn't fulfilled being at home full-time, but I had no idea where I could ever be employed, either.

My fears and frustrations erupted one night in pent-up, hot fury. The person I took it out on was my husband who, I had decided, was living the ungrateful life of a king.

The trigger had been that we'd gotten our annual Social Security notices predicting what we could expect to receive when we hit retirement age. While Haywood had always had a salary, and had had Social Security deductions and retirement benefits accruing every year since we got married, I hadn't built up anything. My expected Social Security payout was zero and my retirement savings were practically non-existent. Feeling hopeless about having any career, and seeing in black-and-white what my long days, sleepless nights and non-stop service to my family was going to result in—at least in this forum—started a conflagration.

"Looks like I'm going to be poor when I'm old," I threw out bitterly as we went to bed. I was starting to sound like Bayard, but while his prompt had been a wallet, mine was the U.S. mail.

Haywood turned to look at me. "What are you talking about?"

"Did it ever occur to you that I'm providing an unpaid service to you and the kids that I'm not getting compensated for?"

He rolled his eyes. This was not a new fight. "C, I've told you that whatever is mine is yours," he said wearily. "I'm sorry we never set up an IRA for you, but you have to learn to look out for yourself too. I can't do everything." That last statement was like waving a red flag in front of a bull.

"How can I do that when *I'm* the one taking care of everything? Isn't there anything you can do to make my life easier? Did it ever occur to you that when you leave for work every morning, and you know that your children are being taken care of by their mother, I've given you a priceless gift of peace of mind?"

I continued in a hot rush. "Do you realize what a sacrifice I've made for you and your career? Do you know that I can't even leave the house for a few hours without worrying what is happening here or who is with my children? You just assume that everything will get done every day, that the kids will be safe, that they will get where they need to go, and that the house will be taken care of all day when you walk out of here in the morning. In case you hadn't figured it out, I'm the person making it possible for you to have the life you're living. You can do anything you want... you can pursue any profession you dream of, travel anywhere on a moment's notice, and stay out late without worrying about who is feeding your children or putting them to bed. Why? Because you have an unpaid domestic laborer as a wife!"

Haywood was silent. He knew there was truth in what I was saying, but didn't know how to end the argument peacefully. His usual comeback, "I do more than most husbands," wasn't going to fly tonight because it always made me angry to hear that he was a saint compared to every other man on the planet.

"You can do whatever you want too" he finally offered. "I've always said that I'll support you in anything you want to do."

"How about a 'thank you' every now and then?" Now I was on a roll. "Can you thank me for always being the one to take the kids to amusement parks with their teams and classes? Someone has to go, and you refuse because you get sick on rides. So I'm the one who spends hours and hours driving to and from these things. Do you think it's how I always want to spend my free time? Someone has to find and research summer camps. You seem to think that they just magically appear on a calendar because they are supposed to be there. You don't even realize how far in advance you have to apply for them and how much time it takes to find and arrange them, and then do all of that driving too."

I gestured angrily towards his closet. "What about your shirts?" You expect me to drop them off and pick them up, but what errands do you do for me? Have you ever even *asked* if you can pick up something for me? And do you think that groceries are teleported from the store and into our refrigerator by Star Trek beams?"

Thankfully, I ran out of steam and the argument ended, but without resolution. I never get anywhere when I go into a frenzy like this. I had to solve this particular dilemma for myself, but I didn't know how. I finally faced it head-on when my desire to feel better outweighed my fears about doing something about it.

✳ ✳ ✳ ✳ ✳ ✳ ✳ ✳

WHEN BAYARD ENTERED kindergarten, I finally had six free hours a day when all three were in school between September and June. It felt like the right time to take action and consider my options. My sessions with Shep began to revolve around trying to make sense of what I could do with myself during the hours I did have, despite knowing that I'd still likely face disruptions that would require my attention. Samantha and I had gotten our black belts earlier that year too, so I had no excuse not to focus exclusively on finding a way to work.

"How about tutoring people in writing?" Shep threw out ideas regularly. I frowned. "I could do it, but I don't think it's really my calling," I countered.

"You'd be a great therapist," he often noted, encouraging me to look into local programs that would result in a Master's in Social Work or a degree as a Licensed Practical Counselor. I thought long and hard about this suggestion, and agreed that while I might be good at it, I didn't want to make a professional life that revolved around listening to people's miseries. I'd finally walked away from the eating disorder field because I'd felt spent by the energy it required to maintain empathy, and was unable to shake off some of the sad situations I heard about. Perhaps I feel things too deeply?

We went around and around for months. Teaching piano? No. Writing speeches for a politician? No. Everything was a no... nothing felt right to me. My frustration continued to rise.

Then one day Shep greeted me with some handouts he'd picked up at a weekend workshop for therapists. The burgeoning field of life coaching was attracting therapists who wanted to transform their practices so they could work with people in a more positive and proactive way, and although it wasn't something Shep wanted to pursue, he saw my name written all over it. "You could do this," he said simply, leaning forward and handing me the information. "You don't have to be a therapist to do it; lots of people like you are doing it because of their backgrounds in helping others in some way. You qualify."

As I perused the handouts and he expressed confidence in my ability to become a coach, I felt like I'd come home. "Right way!" was flashing brightly. I had found my calling.

＊ ＊ ＊ ＊ ＊ ＊ ＊ ＊

ONE OF THE MOST common things you hear professional life and executive coaches say is that when they found the profession of coaching, they realized that they'd been doing it for years, but hadn't known what to call it. That was exactly my sentiment because, since *My Name is Caroline* was published, I'd often found myself in the position of encouraging people to believe in themselves and to go after the life they most wanted instead of settling for less than they deserved. One of the main lessons I'd learned from my eating disorder was that life is precious, and that the people who achieve lives of purpose and meaning are the ones who set their sights high and refuse to quit when the going gets tough.

My research yielded information about why coaching was exploding while other self-help professions were not. Coaching started with the premise that clients are whole, healthy and functioning, and that the coaching relationship is about partnering with a client to help identify and accomplish meaningful goals. Therapy, on the other hand, started with the premise that the client is broken and fits a diagnosis of some type that requires addressing weaknesses or deficits.

As I dug more deeply into coaching and how to get the credentials needed to actually call myself a coach, I found out that the field was somewhat unregulated, but that certain types of training were more credible than others. Also, it was a field that operated quite often in a virtual way, with both the training and coaching occurring on the internet and over the telephone. This was the perfect solution to my fragmented schedule. Not only could I get the training and supervision I required to enter the field, I could probably also work from home and fit clients around my children's lives.

I immediately signed up for a program called "CoachU" that would take me through at least 120 hours of virtual training from credentialed coaches, and I joined the International Coach Federation, the acknowledged leader in organizing and credentialing coaches. I could see that there were many challenges to the field, including the accurate criticism that anyone could call themselves a coach with zero training, and that there was no shared body of literature that would create a set of consistent standards around the world. But it was also clear that when coaching was done in a professional manner, clients from the corporate world and the private sector would be eager to take advantage of our services.

I plunged happily into this world, and quickly hired my own coach so that I could have guidance and accountability to create my own practice. It wasn't long before I had people calling me who had read *My Name is Caro-*

*line*, and wanted to know if I could coach them on overcoming their eating disorders. Working with people who had active diagnoses, like bulimia, was frowned upon within the coaching community, but there were times when therapists encouraged me to work with their clients so that I could remain focused on helping with day-to-day follow-through and life goals, while they worked on the therapeutic issues that were better designed for their training.

My days became the hybrid approach to being a working parent that I had hoped I could find. When my children left for school in the morning, I got busy with CoachU classes and clients, but by 3 p.m., I was back to being a mother. In a stroke of luck, we learned about a housekeeper who wanted to be sponsored for a green card and whose hours and rates were so flexible that she fit our needs perfectly. Having her in our house most days, while I pursued my career in my office on the top floor, was the perfect solution. If there was an emergency, I had two pairs of hands to help with the juggling, and I was able to slip in and out of my roles more easily.

Although I began by working with people who had found me through my books, I began to see that my calling was really helping people set and accomplish goals that would transform their lives. While these goals could include overcoming an eating disorder, more often I began to get clients who wanted to make a big career shift, pursue a lifelong ambition that they were obsessing about, or to just take control of their lives by creating a five-year plan. They also wanted to refine their purpose and be compelled to live in accord with it. I remembered Donny saying that her life had felt meaningless just before she died, and I wish I could have had these types of discussions with her because it might have helped her to see how much she mattered to her grandchildren, and how many of her positive behaviors had created a template for me.

In addition to my CoachU training, I began to study voraciously in the areas of human motivation, sport psychology, and goal setting. I took extra courses and seminars to beef up my understanding of how to be effective in the areas of change and emotional growth, but I soon became aware of the fact that I longed for some rigorous training that would do two things: give me some seriously challenging educational resources, and help combat the perception that coaching was a lightweight profession with poorly-trained practitioners.

I began to clip articles about programs that Fortune 500 companies used to assist employees in setting goals and maintaining habit change. Over and over, I ran into mentions of "the Corporate Athlete" program run by Dr. Jim Loehr in Orlando, Florida, a frequent destination for top executives who were being groomed for leadership positions or who were already running major initiatives and corporations. The center was run on the principles set out in Loehr's best-selling book, *The Power of Full Engagement*, which I inhaled in one sitting. The book advocated ways to live professional lives modeled on the habits of successful athletes, and it cited lots of studies to support its claims, not just anecdotes.

In October 2004, I decided to put myself through the program on my own dime to see what I could learn that would give me new skills to make me a better coach. After 2 ½ days of learning about interval training for the body and mind, how to design a mission statement, and how to work at maximum effectiveness, I left with some new ideas, but I wanted more than the program could offer in such a short time.

I started to think harder about taking Shep's advice about going to school for therapy training. At least I'd be in a profession that had clear standards and practices undergirded with empirical evidence if I joined the ranks of counselors. To give this thinking a try, I visited the Albert Ellis School in Rational Emotive Behavior Therapy in New York City for some one-day workshops, and I fell in love with the approach. Ellis' work, which had resulted in some of the most profound shifts in therapeutic approaches in the 20th century, was based on deliberately altering one's thinking so that behavior change followed, and its simple models leant themselves well to a proactive coaching approach. There was much I could borrow from this training that would help me in coaching, so I applied for their introductory program and prepared for a new chapter in my life.

* * * * * * * *

Since early 2000, I'd been working with one of the country's top executive coaches, Judy Feld, whose guidance had been invaluable in the creation and growth of my practice. In the five years of our work together, I'd gone from no clients to dozens, I'd successfully run coaching groups in teleseminars, and I'd completed my first coaching credential. She was expensive, but I'd wanted to be mentored by the best person I could afford, and it couldn't hurt that she was elected president of the International Coach Federation during our time together, which gave me an even better window into the problems and opportunities facing coaches.

Judy understood my desire to go deeper in my training, but when she heard that I'd applied for the Albert Ellis training, she offered an alternative.

"The University of Pennsylvania is starting a Master's program in Applied Positive Psychology this fall," she noted. "Marty Seligman is running it, and it would give you the best of all possible worlds if you got in. It's an Ivy League school with an academic approach to learning and positive psychology, so you'd get the education you want, and you'd also be able to dig deeper into the tools of change that Seligman has come up with."

Judy was in a position to know a lot about positive psychology because she'd been one of the people behind launching Marty's Authentic Happiness Coaching program, which had been the most successful virtual education ever launched in our field. In less than two years, thousands of professionals had signed up for his six-month telephone training on the fundamentals of the science of happiness. Because coaching was supposed to focus on helping "whole and healthy" people to flourish and not to assist depressed people who needed therapy, this scientific training had drawn a lot of enthusiasm and attention from around the world.

I knew Seligman's work because I had read and was using his books, *Learned Optimism* and *Authentic Happiness*, in my work, but I hadn't heard about the master's program. "Maybe I should just sign up for the telephone training first, to see what I think," I responded.

"You can't... it's over. Marty has decided to put all of his energy and time into creating a more in-depth program at Penn, and that's the only place I'm aware of where you can actually go and learn this type of stuff. Go read the *Time* magazine issue on Positive Psychology that just came out. You'll see what I'm talking about."

I couldn't get my hands on the magazine fast enough. I had a funny feeling of *déjà vu* when I saw it. On the front was a huge yellow smiley face, along with a headline about how the new science of positive psychology was changing the world. It was the same smiley face I'd seen in the early 1990s, touting the efficacy of Prozac. I hoped that this time the smile portended something better for me.

As I pored through article after article about this new field that was changing medicine, psychology, consulting and even teaching, I got more and more excited. And then I came to the page where my "Right Way!" neon sign lit up in ways it hadn't since 17 years ago when I woke up with the certainty that I was going to have a baby.

"The University of Pennsylvania will be accepting 34 men and women into its inaugural Master's degree in applied positive psychology...."

I stopped breathing as I continued to read the article detailing the extensive education accepted students would receive starting in just a few short months. I had to go. I just *had* to go. Every fiber of my body and brain was screaming "Right Way!" and I didn't think I'd ever been surer of anything in my life. If it took my last dollar and dying breath, I had to get into that class and mortgage my soul to pay for it. I knew, deep down, that it would change my life.

I scrambled. The deadline for applications wasn't far off, and I had to get my hands on things I'd never seen before, like my transcript from Harvard. I also had to get two letters of recommendation supporting my professional experience and ability to complete the workload during the year-long program. Thank goodness I'd created a career of some kind, I thought ruefully, because without it I wouldn't have even been considered. Shep and Judy offered to write the letters I needed, so I set about assembling my application packet.

The questions on the application were straightforward. I was asked to describe myself, why I wanted to come to Penn, and what I anticipated I would add to my profession as a result of getting this particular master's degree. I also wrote about my desire to bring more science to the coaching field so that people who wanted a more in-depth study of theories and research could build their practices with a new type of credibility.

I wondered if I'd made a strong enough case for myself when I was done, so I decided to take a risk and add one more question to the application.

"You didn't ask specifically why you should take me, so I wanted to give you ten reasons why I'd be a great member of this first class," I wrote. I came up with what I hoped were nine compelling points, and then I thought about the last one and decided to go for it. "Because I'm fun!"

I was nervous as I sealed up the huge packet of information and sent it in. It would be several months before I learned anything, so I had no choice except to wait.

\* \* \* \* \* \* \* \*

"MOM, YOU GOT a call from the University of Pennsylvania!" Samantha greeted me at the door in early July with a smile on her face. "You have to call back... they didn't leave a message."

Uh oh. It was going to be bad news, I thought. For months after submitting my application, I'd heard nothing, and then in June I'd had a phone interview with James Pawelski and his assistant, Debbie Swick, to narrow down the field of candidates. Although I thought the interview had gone well, it had ended with Debbie's final question: "What's the biggest failure you've ever experienced?"

Renewal's bankruptcy still haunted me as the biggest failure I'd ever had. The pain of losing my pride, our money, our friends' money, and our dreams of creating long-term healing and change for eating disorder sufferers had never really gone away. In fact, I'd recently gotten an email that had unexpectedly brought it all back. The chief financial officer of Standard Healthtrust, whose name I hadn't thought of in fifteen years, had written out of the blue and asked me for help in finding an eating disorder treatment center for his daughter's best friend. The irony that this man, whose company had pulled the plug on our dream, was reaching out to me for help to find a center just like Renewal wasn't lost on me.

Debbie and James thanked me for my time, but I wished we'd ended on something more positive than talking about Renewal. They hadn't mentioned my added application question. Maybe it had been too risky, I worried as we hung up. I also began to worry that the program was too disorganized to get off the ground. We'd been told that acceptances would go out in May, but here we were in mid-summer with no word yet. Maybe the program was too cutting-edge for the Ivies.

I checked Caller I.D. for the number and sat down for the bad news. The people who'd actually gotten in had probably been told weeks earlier so they could plan their fall schedules.

Debbie Swick answered her phone. "Congratulations, Caroline! You've been admitted to our first MAPP class!"

I went numb. I had gotten in? They wanted me? It was too much good news all at once. Samantha was staring at me, trying to read my face.

"Did you get in?" she mouthed.

I nodded.

"Yes!" She ran around fist-pumping. "Mom got into Penn! Mom got into Penn! She's going to school! Yay!"

Her enthusiasm was contagious. I hung up and hugged her. "I did it! I got in!"

Although I knew change was about to occur in my life in multiple ways, little did I know that my entire way of thinking, living and working was going to be profoundly altered as a result of my admission to MAPP. And the biggest surprise was that it gave me a new language and comprehension of how and why my eating disorder recovery had proven to be so durable over so many years.

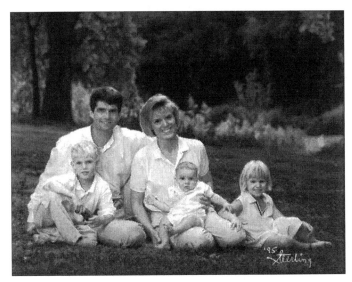

IN AUGUST 1995, WE POSED AS A FAMILY OF FIVE AT THE
NEIGHBORHOOD PARK WHERE MY GRANDMOTHER HAD
TAUGHT ME TO RIDE MY BIKE 30 YEARS EARLIER.
PHOTOGRAPH: STERLING PHOTOGRAPHY

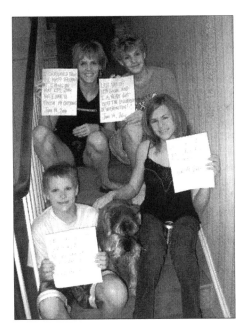

FIRST AND LAST DAYS: IN SEPTEMBER 2005,
I JOINED THE CHILDREN AND OUR DOG,
SPLASH, ON OUR FRONT STEPS WHERE WE
HELD UP OUR SIGNS ANNOUNCING THAT WE
WERE ALL GOING BACK TO SCHOOL SOON.

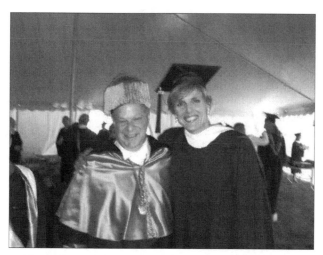

MARTY SELIGMAN, KNOWN AS "THE FATHER OF POSITIVE PSYCHOLOGY," ENCOURAGED ME TO WRITE MY CAPSTONE PROJECT ON THE INTERSECTION OF GOAL-SETTING THEORY WITH THE SCIENCE OF HAPPINESS, WHICH LATER BECAME THE BEST-SELLING BOOK, "CREATING YOUR BEST LIFE."

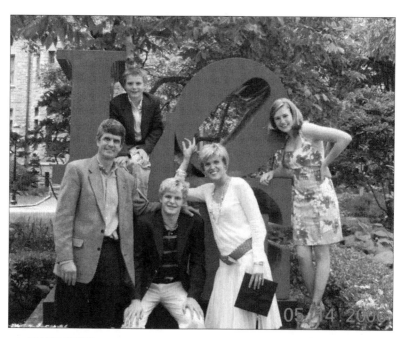

IN MAY 2006, MY FAMILY JOINED ME AT THE INFAMOUS "LOVE" STATUE ON THE CAMPUS OF THE UNIVERSITY OF PENNSYLVANIA. LATER THAT DAY I WAS ONE OF THE FIRST 34 PEOPLE IN THE WORLD TO EARN A MASTER OF APPLIED POSITIVE PSYCHOLOGY DEGREE

## CHAPTER TWENTY THREE
## ENDINGS AND BEGINNINGS

When Haywood was in pre-school, I began a tradition of having the children hold up signs stating that it was the first or last day of school. Accordingly, every September and June, give or take a few weeks, they dutifully lined up on our entrance hall staircase holding white poster boards announcing the grade they were entering or leaving, as well as the day. When Haywood was ten he achieved a big swimming goal, so a Standard Schnauzer puppy named Splash entered the family, and he too joined the fun by perching on a step on the appointed time and day, never missing a picture.

My scrapbook album documenting these transitions, called "Beginnings and Endings," expanded by at least two pictures every year, so it was easy to track how the children were changing in big and small ways as they grew up. In the early years, there were a lot of toothless grins and outfits that I'd picked out, which morphed into hairstyles and clothes that they chose for themselves. Haywood's hair became more and more fluorescent as the chlorine in the pools left its mark. Samantha's spurts in growth were particularly noticeable, as she needed more and more room to stretch out her endless legs that extended until she hit almost six feet. Bayard's changes were in line with his tendency to do everything early; in his kindergarten picture he possessed the mature face and look of a high school senior, so in subsequent years he just looked like a different version of that man, give or take a few teeth or rows of braces.

It only seemed fitting then, that I joined the lineup in September 2005. I nestled among the children and held up my sign stating that I was returning to the University of Pennsylvania for a Master's degree in Applied Positive Psychology. "Wish me luck," I added at the bottom of the sign.

Although I possessed a good educational pedigree and had always found that learning environments were my favorite place to be, I really didn't have a sense of what awaited me, so I thought a little bit of luck couldn't hurt. I knew there would be lots of reading and monthly papers, but those had always come easily to me, so I wondered more about the other parts. What would my classmates be like? Would they like me? Would I find some new friends who might stand the test of time once the program was over? Did people take written notes in class anymore, or was it all electronic note-taking? Would I get what I went there to find? Would it make me happier? Would it be worth the investment of time and money?

I also wondered what I would wear in a collegiate setting that wouldn't reek of being a middle-aged mommy, so I enlisted Samantha's help as I opened a huge suitcase and prepared myself for Immersion Week—a five-day, dawn to dusk set of classes that would introduce us to many of the leaders in the Positive Psychology field, both in person and through their writings. My own college years had been at the height of my eating disorder, so all I remembered wearing then were sweat suits, overalls and other shapeless, athletic outfits that I used to hide myself. I'd obviously moved on from that look, but the pickings were still slim as I surveyed my closet because clothing hadn't been high on my investment list as the kids were growing up. Everything seemed to fit from year to year, too, so there was never a reason to shop. Samantha determined that a few peasant skirts, blouses, sandals, jeans and shirts would do the trick, so I packed those, then threw in a lot of other stuff, just in case.

One of my biggest logistical worries about leaving town for a five-day stretch was successfully addressed the day before my departure when Haywood came home triumphantly with his driver's license. His father had taken him to the Motor Vehicle Administration while I got myself ready, and unlike many of his peers, he had actually passed the test on the first try, which meant that he could transport himself from now on to the 4:45 am and 3:30 pm swim practices he attended every day. For the other two kids, I'd lined up some supportive friends, who were only too willing to help me with my normal daily quota of carpools, pickups and other activities. I was actually one of several moms who were returning to school to get advanced degrees in subjects ranging from interior design to special education teaching, so we were all banding together when the need arose for coverage, helping each other through the bumpy transition so that no one's needs were neglected.

Haywood had always been an involved father when he could be, and was particularly engaged in the children's weekend sports commitments, but he'd never been a single father for five days, so I knew he was probably going to miss my presence more than anyone in the house. In some ways, I thought, this might be good because he'd become so accustomed to leaving town whenever he needed to, or simply attending to his own affairs and work needs all day, that he'd lost sight of how I actually spent my days, and how much juggling I was doing to keep both the family and my own work going.

My decision to go back to school wasn't popular within our extended families, which made it more challenging for both of us on some levels, particularly because the criticism of me was so petty. Haywood's parents privately voiced their unhappiness about my decision to return to school to him on many occasions, wondering why I'd made his life harder by adding any household chores to his load. I also occasionally heard Haywood on the phone with them, defending the fact that I had every right to go back to school, given how much I'd done in service to the family for so many years, and that it wasn't even a financial burden on us (in an incredibly kind gesture, my brother decided to pass along some of the financial help he'd received over the years from my parents, and he underwrote my entire year). Haywood's parents seemed to have forgotten that I was the one who had worked and supported us while their son went through law school and business school, but I suspected that much of their beef was just that they honestly believed that I wasn't a good mother if I did anything that wasn't exclusively childcare or housekeeping. My own mother was no better; she made fun of the degree when she learned I'd been admitted, saying that a one-year Master's degree had to simply be Penn's effort at fundraising, and not a *bona fide* educational opportunity.

Nevertheless, I was excited to leave on September 3rd, 2005, knowing that the next year of my life would not only be life-changing in one way or another, it would also be my way of revisiting and healing my regrets about the opportunities I'd missed at Harvard while my eating disorder ruled my life. This time, I was going to get the educational thing right and make it count.

* * * * * * * *

THE UNIVERSITY OF PENNSYLVANIA is in Philadelphia, just over the Schuykill River and not far from the historic downtown, which still houses the Liberty Bell and buildings where some of our country's most important founding moments occurred. The university's buildings are reminiscent of what I remembered from Harvard, but I still found myself so awestruck at the fact that I was starting classes at an Ivy League school in my mid-forties that I had to pull off to the side of the street to collect myself when I glimpsed an arch spanning Walnut Street that said "The University of Pennsylvania." I fumbled for my camera like a star-struck tourist, then collected myself before entering Huntsman Hall for our class's welcoming session with Marty Seligman and the program's head, James Pawelski.

From the moment I sat down in a chair in the back row and began to listen to Marty and other leaders in the field of psychology, including Ray Fowler, Barry Schwartz and Chris Peterson, I was certain that this was exactly where I was supposed to be. "Right Way!" could not have been more accurate about foretelling the power of this new chapter of my life. Here was the education I'd been looking for, and every word spoken resonated with me on two levels—first as a person, and second as a professional. I'd found a new home.

One of the most galvanizing moments of the week occurred when Barbara Fredrickson spoke about her work with the Positivity Ratio, and how the highest-functioning marriages, work teams and relationships all operated over the ratio of three to one: three positive comments or interactions for one negative. The most optimal ratio was five to one, and Barb emphasized how important it was that we take charge of our lives either by raising the positives or reducing the negatives so that we could create flourishing environments wherever we were.

As Barb spoke, I saw my life as a mother flashing before my eyes. Bayard and Samantha were generally easier to parent because they usually followed directions and didn't get into trouble, but my relationship with my oldest son had become very hard in recent years. Our occasional screaming matches were epic in the house. Headstrong, impulsive and moody, Haywood was a carbon copy of me, which meant that we often butted heads, especially because I had fallen into being the disciplinarian of the children while Haywood preferred to be the guy who came home at the end of the day to watch movies, play baseball or do other fun activities. It was easy to see how my ratio with my younger children was probably in the right zone, but I wondered if my ratio with my oldest was closer to one-to-one, which Barb was saying would result in downward spirals of negativity that boded ill for everyone involved.

As Barb shared her mathematical formulas and research with our class, I mused sadly about how I often led with criticism and anger when Haywood challenged my authority instead of trying to find something positive to say before we tangled. Already, I had a takeaway from this program that I knew was going to make my life richer, and although I couldn't go anywhere in that moment, I found myself wanting to leave Penn immediately to go home and work on righting the ratio in my relationship with my oldest son. A picture snapped of me and some of my classmates surrounding Barb after she finished shows me just staring up at her, speechless, amazed that

I'd just been given a tool that not only made sense to me, but there was real evidence that it actually worked and its application in multiple ways was crystal-clear to me.

My reaction to Barb's lecture was repeated over and over during the five days as I learned about Well Being Theory, "flow," the "paradox of choice," "positive interventions," global well-being measures, character strength research, and much more. I don't often find myself at a loss for words but when I called home late at night from Penn to share my day, I often had no ability to describe my reactions to what I was learning. One night, flat on my back and staring at the ceiling of my hotel room, I said in exhaustion to my husband, "I feel like my brain is an unformatted computer disk and I'm taking in so much information that nothing is fitting anywhere. I'm flooded."

Our class was composed of 33 other men and women from multiple occupations and countries, all of whom shared a pioneer's passion to learn about this exciting new science of happiness although no role models existed for how to actually use the degree when we were done. Dave Shearon, a lawyer from Tennessee whom I nicknamed Socrates for his long questions and oratorical skills, stopped our class cold one day when he drawled, "So what the hell are we when we're done here? What is a MAPP, anyway?" Dozens of adult men and women ranging in age from 22 to 60 looked to the front of the room for guidance.

Marty's answer was that he wanted us to take the research we'd be learning all year and "apply" it to our respective fields so that we could bring more emotional flourishing to teaching, law, financial services, coaching, business, politics, entrepreneurial activities, consulting, sport psychology, and the other professions represented in the class. As he spoke, I already knew that applying the positivity ratio research to my own life would be interesting, and I was looking forward to how I'd be using that and other theories in new ways in my coaching practice. We could help to "increase the tonnage of happiness" in the world if we were creative and persistent in this task, he counseled. He would leave it up to us to figure out how to do that, but he told us that he felt certain he was unleashing a new wave of change by filling our brains with the work of esteemed researchers and encouraging us to think outside the box around its application. "This will never be just a psychology degree," he passionately explained. "This is an *applied* psychology degree, and my goal is for you to become a bridge from academia to the real world by seeing how this research can be used for meaningful change."

For this mission, which he often said felt like the most important undertaking of his life, he'd selected some of the most fascinating people I'd met in a long time, and all of us found ourselves engaging in endless conversations before and after classes, over meals, and late into the night. Befriending the comedian Yakov Smirnoff, whom I originally mistook for the singer Cat Stevens (he later told me that he wasn't offended because he had no idea who Cat Stevens was), was just one of the unexpected benefits of being in the program. His mission was unusual: he wanted to learn how to use laughter to enhance happiness among couples because he said that when he heard laughter between his parents when he was growing up in Russia, he knew there was love in the room regardless of how poor they were.

This was the intoxicating atmosphere in which I found myself. I couldn't remember a time since Harvard when I'd been around so many bright, curious and diverse people from all over the world whose level of conversational skills was so high and whose interests were so varied that I couldn't do something as simple as go to the bathroom without learning about microfinance while washing my hands. Although my circle of friends at home wasn't composed of slackers, spending most of my days and years since college primarily raising children had reduced the quality of many conversations to discussions of necessity: Where do you need to be and at what time? Who do you want to do a play date with? What would you like for dinner? Did you finish your homework? Rarely had I enjoyed extended, in-depth discussions with anyone about ideas that truly engaged my brain for at least fifteen years, and I found myself as hungry for that stimulation as I'd once been for food.

Although I entered the program with a certain amount of cockiness about my writing abilities, the first assignment exposed the rustiness of my brain and analytical skills. On the surface, it looked simple: "Read and synthesize the materials relating to positive interventions from several historical periods and come up with your own theory of what a positive intervention is."

I understood the words, but suddenly had no idea how to actually go about doing the assignment. Sitting in the borrowed office of one of my friends on a weekend afternoon, I felt my head start to swim, and I had the surprising panicky reaction of wanting to cry. I put my head down on the desk where the materials were spread out and tried to think of how I was going to do this little three-page paper. I'd done something like this hundreds of times in my life, and had written many newspaper stories on deadline, but I hadn't actually exercised this type of approach to my thoughts in decades so I was momentarily lost. After a minute of feeling emotionally hijacked, I sat up, reminded myself that if I'd done it before I could do it again, and forced myself to begin to read. Eight hours later, the sun down, I emerged wearily from the office with my first draft, stunned at how much effort it had taken. This was going to be a lot harder than I had anticipated.

The family had mixed reactions to my new love for what I was learning. On the plus side, they liked the fact that I had homework because that made me one of them. They hadn't ever heard some of the words I began to throw around like "self-efficacy" and "self-regulation," and they wanted to know more about the people I was meeting and where they were from. One of my classmates, Sulynn Choong, had relocated from Malaysia for one year to be in the program, leaving her young daughter behind with her husband and relatives, which emphasized to my family that my education was unusual enough that people were willing to go to great lengths to be there. And Sulynn wasn't the only one traveling great distances every single month to be exposed to the learning; Angus Skinner came from Scotland and Juan Williams from Switzerland. John Yeager was there on behalf of the Culver Academy in Indiana, which was investing heavily in creating a character education program with John at its head, and Gloria Park had abandoned her pursuit of a PhD in sport psychology to add this knowledge to her career before going back to finish her other degree.

On the other hand, my children weren't accustomed to having me away every month for four days, and things dropped through the cracks at those times. Essentials like milk didn't get replenished when they ran out, no one was around to bail them out if homework was forgotten at home, and there wasn't a welcoming presence when they returned home from school every day, other than the dog and an occasional appearance from our part-time housekeeper. Although I missed being that mom, there was no hiding the fact that I felt like I was on fire in every way, emotionally, physically and spiritually. Much like I'd felt when I left my infant son to appear on "To Tell the Truth" in 1990, fifteen years later I was experiencing a surge of joy and relief that I could walk out of my house for a few days and not be responsible for a myriad of mind-numbing details that I'd grown weary of handling, and that I could do something that was just for me for hours at a time. Once, my older son commented as I walked back in from another four days of positive psychology infusion: "You're so much happier when you come back from Penn. Maybe you should just move there."

Indeed, it was impossible not to notice, as the months went on, that I was being transformed from the inside out. Every single day I was in class or reading new research on awe, elevation, gratitude, social capital, and character strengths, I learned about and later experimented with ways to enhance my own life and well-being while also bringing new tools to my coaching practice that were instantly benefiting my clients too. Within weeks of starting the program I was sharing my assignments and the rationale behind them with some of the clients I worked with who were curious about the topics, as well as discussing with them the Positivity Ratio and how to track events in their own lives to get a sense of whether or not they were languishing or flourishing. In this way, I was clearly getting many of the benefits I had hoped to get from the master's program.

What I wasn't prepared for as part of my MAPP year, however, was that so much of what I'd done to deal with my bulimia and get into long-term recovery was now being explained to me with psychological theories and research from the world of goal-setting, positive psychology, sport psychology, and human motivation. Every month yielded a new Eureka moment that had the impact of helping me understand how I had made it into middle-age without relapse, always finding ways to bounce back from setbacks that had led others to return to self-destructive behavior.

I began to see how positive psychology and the concept of taking charge of our own emotional flourishing could have a place in the addiction treatment world because so much of it dovetailed with what I'd had to learn the hard way through trial and error. I wondered how much more quickly I might have made progress if I'd known about the differences between being in authentic "flow"—when time stands still because you are engaging in a positive challenge where the task exceeds your abilities—versus "junk flow," which I identified as time standing still when I went into my bulimic fugue state for hours. Substituting one for the other might have been a healthy, early intervention on my behavior.

In my therapy sessions with Kathleen, she had mentioned that I needed to see myself as someone who possessed a collection of strengths that should be acknowledged and used to enhance confidence and change, instead of focusing on my weaknesses or failures, like Renewal's bankruptcy. Now I heard this same call to action as part of the foundational definition of positive psychology, which was explained as the study of what was good and worthy of replication, and that also enhanced individual and group flourishing.

An early assignment called for us to take the VIA (Values in Action) Strengths test, which identified our top five character strengths out of 24 universally admired traits, and to write about a time when all of our top strengths were being used and we were "at our best." When I finished the thirty-minute test, I was eager to see what it discerned, but was initially surprised by my lineup. "The ability to love others and be loved back," led the list, followed by "creativity," "zest," "wisdom" and "bravery." I didn't immediately identify with being a wise, brave and loving person, but in a flash I knew exactly what my "Me at My Best" essay would be about.

"When I wrote my first book, *My Name is Caroline*," I began my paper, "I now see that I was at my best, even though the book was about me at my worst." Although I'd talked about honoring my strengths in therapy, doing this assignment crystallized the importance of the concept because I matched the idea of having unique abilities with a specific occurrence, plus I had the added benefit of a test telling me exactly what my top strengths were instead of me guessing what they were. I went on to say that my ability to love myself enough to fight for my life, as well as my love for others whom I wanted to benefit from my story, was how I saw my first strength playing out in the writing of the book. Second, I had to be creative to tell a story in such a way that people wanted to read it. Third, it was my zest and love for life that gave me the oomph to even want recovery or have the energy and passion to pursue it. The wisdom and bravery were manifested by being among the first to tell the raw tale of a tough period in my life, but also to show how much richer my life was as the result of bottoming out at such a young age.

As I continued to muse on these thoughts, I recalled multiple times when I had approached a task in a creative way, or with boldness, and been successful in that endeavor. I could see how those strengths, and especially zest, had been present when I connected with clients on the phone, or gave a speech that resulted in the feedback that people felt energized by my encouraging words and my presence. When I led with my best traits, I gave myself a better chance at being received well by others. Much of the sadness that pervaded my eating disorder years had been when I tried to be something I wasn't. What if I'd known my strengths as a young teen, and had seen those as a way to build my confidence rather than always thinking that I had to focus on what was wrong with me?

One of the key concepts we learned during Immersion Week was about how the introduction of "positive interventions"—voluntary shifts in behavior or thinking—could help us be in a flourishing place, and specifically over the 3:1 ratio. Among the interventions that had been studied and found to reliably improve mood were exercise, journal writing, the practice of gratitude, altruistic behavior, having a forgiving attitude, meditation, and pursuing valued goals. My self-help group for recovering overeaters had encouraged most of these behaviors, underscored with slogans like, "Have an attitude of gratitude," "Take it easy," and "You can't keep what you don't give away." We had also been encouraged to write down our progress through the steps, and to do a practice of making amends and asking for forgiveness from those we had wronged. Those actions included the premise that we needed to forgive ourselves, as well. Without even knowing it, I had stumbled into a positive psychology boot camp of sorts in 1984 that had clearly caused me to flourish while helping me put the brakes on my self-destructive behavior.

This idea that putting myself into a positive frame of mind must have played some type of role in ultimately achieving abstinence from bulimia was cemented in our second month of the program, and it caused me to rethink everything I was doing with my coaching clients. We were assigned a brand-new report authored by three of the leading researchers in the positive psychology field that summarized all the findings to date on success. It said that regardless of the domain, people who achieved any type of success did so by first being in a positive emotional state. Put simply, whether the goal was around salary, friendship, health, or any other desirable outcome, the evidence was that happy people were overwhelmingly more likely to get what they wanted than people who were in a less desirable emotional place. People don't become happy because they are successful; they become successful because they are happy first. This was a revolutionary concept for me, and certainly one that I'd never heard before.

Similar to the moment when I heard about the Positivity Ratio, while reading this research I couldn't stop thinking about my own life because it explained so much of what had puzzled me while the eating disorder festered. Despite the messages that were pounded into me starting young— achieve goals like good grades, admission to elite colleges, win in sports, have the "right" body—none had made me happy, and this was the first time

I really understood why. I'd been stuck on the "hedonic treadmill," I now learned in MAPP, which would always lead you to adapt to certain external conditions or possessions without ever giving you the lasting pleasure you had thought it would. This was why geographical changes, the purchase of items like ipods and luxury goods, or even the attainment of a huge salary jump never resulted in lasting happiness. The only things that ever appreciated over time, we learned, were experiences we had with other people, and we were encouraged to learn to "savor" those experiences. I also learned that I'd been pursuing "extrinsic" goals—goals set for me by others—which rarely brought happiness if achieved.

So, like a dog chasing its tail, I'd been going in endless circles thinking that the next "win" was going to bring me that emotional fulfillment, a search that had ended in 1984 when I'd despairingly bottomed out with my eating disorder. That low point had led me to slowly attend to the basics in life and find a Higher Power for inner growth, while also giving back to others to keep myself on the right road. My goal wasn't about my body or being a winner any longer; it had become a search for stability and meaning, and "winning" only in the sense that I was becoming the best person I could be. And by making that profound shift, I'd turned the boat in the right direction to stay afloat and continue to sail for another day.

\* \* \* \* \* \* \* \*

IN 1912, MY GRANDFATHER'S brothers, Platt and Ben Adams, jumped to Olympic gold and silver medals at the Stockholm Olympics, becoming the second siblings to go one-two in an Olympic event, with Platt setting the world record in the process. Platt was an especially decorated American athlete, written up in newspapers as one of the best track and field athletes of the first half of the 20th century. There wasn't anything he couldn't do well; the first time he threw the discus he missed the American record by half an inch, and pictures of him with the heralded Jim Thorpe, also a 1912 Olympic athlete, recorded their joint star status. When I was young, my father took us to the New York Athletic Club to see Platt's gold medal on display, so we heard lots of stories growing up about how he'd put together a formidable physical and mental package to get to the sporting heights he'd achieved.

As a result of the family legacy, plus my own competitive spirit—which was proven at MAPP when I took the Gallup Signature Strengths test. I learned that not only was "competitor" my number-one trait—of the 33 other people in my class, none of my classmates even had it in their top five. Clearly, I had an unusual abundance of seeing life as a big competition, much as my great uncles had, but in hindsight, it was obvious that the dark side of "competitor" had resulted in things like bulimia, where competition was taken to an extreme level, and with the wrong goals. Learning to pursue the "right" goals—those I set for myself—in the "right" ways, had occupied my energy ever since I entered recovery.

After my father died and I created my first bucket list in the hope that I'd never leave a stone unturned, the way he'd left his Greek voyage unfulfilled, my coaching practice had naturally tended towards helping people to identify meaningful goals and to craft the plan to get there. I was ideally suited in temperament and strengths to do this, and I brought the passion of knowing how important it was to live each day with gusto because of my recovery, so clients often told me that our work resulted in some of the best progress they'd ever made on hard goals.

I'd sought to learn as much as I could about goal-setting, first through lots of books and seminars, and later through attending the Corporate Athlete Center, but the closest I'd ever come to hearing research about goal accomplishment was the "Harvard Study of 1950" that I found in a number of popular self-help goal books, with basically the same story. The story implied that when the Harvard Class of 1950 had been surveyed thirty years after graduation, those who had written down their goals had been profoundly more successful than graduates who had never written down their goals. I'd seen this anecdote in so many places that I took it for granted that it was true, and I put it on my website as "evidence" that goal-setting worked.

At Penn, though, I was being introduced to real research, with rigorous controls and pages of findings, which whetted my appetite for more solid science to work with in this area. It wasn't long before we had an assignment on "goal setting theory," which apparently was a well-tested theory that had held up in hundreds of studies from the business world in areas like tree-cutting and gadget production. As I read Locke and Latham's research on how they'd assembled their theory decades earlier, I couldn't believe I'd never heard about it a single time during my coach training, despite being told that one of my ethical responsibilities as a coach included being able to help clients set and accomplish goals, as well as track progress. I checked out the entire textbook on goal setting theory from Penn's library and copied every single page so that I had a rock-solid reference with me at all times.

As part of our work at Penn, we were required to come up with a Cap-stone project that would be our own unique study of some aspect of positive psychology. It had to involve the application of what we were learning to a real-world situation. I began to realize that I needed to do something that I hadn't seen done before by any other author.

"Marty, I think I have an idea for my Capstone," I said one night when our entire class gathered at Marty's suburban home near Penn. Although a little hard of hearing, Marty focused intently on me as I spoke because it was a little early to be mentioning this aspect of our year's responsibilities, which wouldn't be due until the following August.

"Tell me what you're thinking."

"I've looked in every bookstore for years for books on goal-setting that have some type of evidence or rigor in them, and I can't find a single one, and certainly one that has any footnotes. They all talk about SMART goals and the Harvard Study of 1950, which I've now learned is an urban legend, and there's nothing about goal setting theory, and there certainly isn't anything that links the studies showing that it's important to be in a positive emotional place to enhance success. I want to write the first book that puts all those theories together."

I went on to say that the bestseller in the field was a book about "The Law of Attraction," and that many coaches worked from that basis with clients, but that I wanted to have a more credible approach. "I want to write a book that can be used in academic settings so that coaches can benefit, but also a popular book so that everyone can learn some of the things I'm learning here that I've never read before. No one has ever done that."

Marty spent a few minutes quizzing me about my idea, and threw out other thoughts for my Capstone, including something that might include health insurance outcomes linking well-being to better health, but I didn't bite. "This book needs to be written, Marty," I insisted. "What if I did my Capstone as a book proposal and two chapters of a new book that could be the basis for what I'm talking about?"

Marty is just as firm and immovable at times as I am, so after throwing out a few more ideas that he hoped would be interesting to me, he sighed and threw up his hands with a smile. "You're going to write the book so it doesn't matter what I say. Go write the book!"

That conversation marked a turning-point in my year because I now felt that I had identified a hole in the coaching and goal setting literature that I could actually plug if I wrote the book in an approachable but solid way, so the rest of the year I operated on two tracks. I did all of my assignments and readings in the areas we were studying—leadership, resilience, grit—but I spent dozens of hours soaking up research in other areas that pertained to the theories I wanted to weave together as part of my book. "Right Way!" flashed constantly as I immersed myself in my new project.

As I did this, part of why I'd come to Penn became clear to me in a new way that I couldn't have known before I got there. Yes, I'd found a program that would help me develop a coaching practice that suited my style, and I also had found a redemptive way to return to school and learn with a clear mind and a healthy body for the first time since 9th grade. But in the process of doing this, I'd also found my purpose. If I could write a book that demonstrated how well-being theory was an integral part of setting goals, and that being able to set and master goals enhances one's self-efficacy (one of the four things that defined a "flourishing" person) I could give people the tools that would show them the bi-directional science of happiness and success, while also helping to educate coaches to learn these important theories that weren't in any of the coaching programs I'd ever encountered. If I could do this, I would have fulfilled the goal that Marty had set before us as part of what he hoped we could accomplish as applied positive psychologists—"increase the tonnage of happiness in the world."

Not only that, it would be my own way of giving meaning to my life. In my first book, I'd talked about my pursuit of my big goal—saving my own life and finding happiness—and now I might be able to pull together a whole new approach to how to set and accomplish any goal, which had to first be addressed by finding happiness. My life had now come full circle with what I was studying and writing about, and it was definitely a "Right Way!" moment.

* * * * * * * *

THE YEAR AT PENN went by too quickly, but the friendships, learning and indelible mark the program left on my life would always be part of me, so it was bittersweet to prepare for graduation in May 2006. In the months leading up to that moment, there had been an international surge of interest in Positive Psychology because Tal ben Shahar, an instructor at Harvard University, was teaching a class in the subject, and it had become the largest, most popular class in the history of the school.

Just before our graduation, several people from my class went to Harvard where we sat in on one of Tal's lectures. I was unprepared for what I saw.

Memorial Hall is one of the largest spaces on the Harvard campus, and that was where Tal's class had been moved to accommodate the hundreds of undergraduates who had gotten into the class. I'd been in this hall several times for some of my survey courses, but the atmosphere had never been like this.

As Tal stepped to the lectern to begin to speak, the room—which had

239

had the normal buzzing of low-pitched voices while we waited—suddenly became eerily quiet. I watched as dozens of rows of young men and women flipped open computers and looked expectantly towards the front of the room. You could have heard a pin drop.

Watching the eagerness in the faces of the students, and seeing how earnestly they took notes and asked questions, was an education in itself. I'd been privileged to hear dozens of brilliant and famous men and women in my time at Harvard, but I'd never seen anyone command this type of respect. After the class, students surrounded us, asking about the Penn program and how it could build on what they were learning. One woman noted, "I've learned a lot in the classes here, but I've never learned so much about myself as a person as I have in Tal's class. This is the first class that I can honestly say has given me tools to make my life better, and I want to keep going."

The media frenzy continued about Tal's class and how Positive Psychology was now spreading to other universities around the world. Penn was already getting more applications for the second year of its MAPP program than they had for the first year, and PhD programs in Positive Psychology were appearing in California and elsewhere. The field I had chosen to study and specialize in was suddenly the hottest game in town, and my gratitude for being part of it was unbounded.

\* \* \* \* \* \* \* \*

ONE OF THE CONCEPTS we learned at Penn was "Peak-End" theory, which posits that we remember events in our lives based on two factors: the best or "peak" moment, and then how it ended. Whether you studied colonoscopies or vacations, people overwhelmingly coded something as a positive experience if both of those moments had been good.

I often thought about that as I went through the year, musing about the ways in which my eating disorder recovery, and healing other emotional scars, had benefitted from this theory. For example, voluntarily returning to play the piano as an adult, after dropping it during my bulimic years, had unwittingly ensured that I was always going to think of piano as a positive, and not with the regrets I'd always lived with. It had instinctively felt like the right thing to do, but learning about the theory had proven why it worked so well. The same was true of swimming. I'd ended my career while the bulimia was in full swing, but after watching Haywood's races for years, I decided to dip my toe back in the water by joining a Masters swim team. Although I did my first 5 am swim practice with the caveat that I was just "trying it out," I fell back in love with the sport that had brought me so much pleasure as a young girl, and I looked forward to the training and competitions instead of seeing them as embarrassing experiences where I didn't want anyone to see my body.

Returning to school as a student who wasn't always looking for the closest bathrooms, and whose brain wasn't constantly foggy from binging and purging or other self-destructive behaviors, was one of the biggest "peak-end" changes I could have created, however. My regrets about lost opportunities at Harvard were completely erased by the extraordinary joy I took from every reading, every class, and every interaction I had with my colleagues in the program in that year. By returning to school, and studying something I was passionate about, I changed how I felt about myself as a student, and crossed off a bucket list goal in the process.

The year ended too soon. Although our Capstone project wasn't due until August 1st, we "walked" with all of the other Penn undergraduates and graduates on a clear, sunny day on the grounds of the University of Pennsylvania in May 2006. I'd taken my family on a tour of the campus in the morning of graduation, showing them the rooms where I'd had my classes, the places I'd eaten so many meals, and the bookstores and benches where I'd engaged in countless conversations that challenged my ways of thinking. We also made the obligatory stop at the famous "Love" statue where we posed for our Christmas card photo.

Not long after, I lined up with my classmates as we wound our way into a tent where family and friends packed the rows of folding chairs. The fact that I was in a cap and gown, surrounded by musical pomp, as over a hundred people stood and clapped for us, was hard to believe. We took our seats on the side of the stage and waited excitedly as we got to the part where we were going to actually get our diplomas.

When I had been an "Adams," I'd usually been in the very front of every line that was alphabetical, but as a "Miller," I had learned to wait my turn. I watched the people ahead of me climb three small steps before they got onto the stage where Marty, James and other Penn dignitaries waited to congratulate us. The line got shorter and shorter, and then it was my turn.

"Caroline Adams Miller!"

James Pawelski called out my name as I literally broke into one of the biggest smiles of my life and danced towards Marty to get my diploma and hug. As I did so, I turned to see my three children and husband stand up together and cheer, "Yay Mom!" I quickly tried to imprint the scene on my memory so that I could call it up whenever I wanted in the future. We'd learned this year that a happy person is also a "savoring" person, and now as an official "applied positive psychologist," I wanted to "apply" the research to myself so that I could always recall this moment with clarity.

I was also moved that my children were on their feet, cheering me on, and that they saw me receiving recognition for something I'd worked so hard to attain. They were accustomed to seeing me cheer for them wherever they were, including sporting events and school graduations, but this was the first time they'd done it for me, and it was sweet.

The ceremony was over too quickly, but the fact that the people who meant the most to me, including my brother, Billy—who had arrived just in time to see me cross the stage—had showed up that day to see my moment of triumph, was exactly what we'd learned all year was at the heart of most happiness: sharing experiences with other people who matter is one of the greatest gifts you can give yourself.

Happiness isn't in things. It's not in status, power, money or geography. It's not in having the "perfect" body, winning a race, or going to Harvard. No... my education this year had decisively taught me what I wished

242

I'd known earlier in my life before I pursued all of the wrong goals. Happiness is in people, love, gratitude, giving, pursuing hard goals, caring, sharing and savoring memories. Happiness had never been "out there" and something to go and find. Happiness had always been in me and around me, and I just had to see it to appreciate it. I knew deep in my heart that the MAPP program had given me—intellectually and emotionally—what I'd been searching for all these years. I was now positively Caroline in every sense of the word.

\* \* \* \* \* \* \* \*

THE REVERBERATIONS from the MAPP program didn't cease for years, and although I thought I'd healed every possible remaining wound that I'd carried around with me from my eating disorder years, I had one last surprise waiting for me in 2008. Just as I gave Sterling Publishing the manuscript for *Creating Your Best Life*, which was the ultimate outgrowth of my Capstone project, I returned to Harvard University for my 25th reunion, which is the reunion where Harvard pulls out all the stops.

I was really fortunate that I had requested my freshman year room, Grays 42, and gotten it, so it was with some nostalgia and apprehension that I mounted the steps to the room where I'd spent my first year of college, praying that my bulimia would magically go away, but scared when it just kept getting worse. Nothing in the room had changed. The wood paneling and hooks where we'd hung our coats and backpacks were still there, and the bedrooms looked smaller than I remembered, especially with the tiny bunk beds pushed up against the walls. The bathroom wasn't updated either, and the huge mirror that greeted you when you entered was the same, but at least now I looked at myself and felt contented, not broken. How often had I stood in front of this mirror, telling myself what a loser I was? Peak-end rule suggested that coming back to this room was another important step.

It turned out that I wasn't the only person who had totally transformed herself in the years between 1983 and 2008. The infamous "red book" that

Harvard issues with biographical updates in the months prior to our gathering is a way to catch up with people we'd lost touch with, as well as to learn more about people we'd never had a chance to meet. These write-ups were interesting, especially because some people had taken enormous risks in pursuing an unconventional career path; they often said they were happier than the people who'd admitted that they'd conformed to what was expected of them. One or two had gone through sex change operations, some had changed their names to suit their passions in life, and a number admitted ruefully to failed marriages, bankrupt businesses, or even ethical violations that had resulted in criminal prosecution. There were also some deaths, including one of my friends from the *Harvard Crimson* newspaper, Connie Laibe, who had succumbed to breast cancer not long after she'd published a heralded book on the soft drink industry, and Andy Sudduth, a rower who'd earned an Olympic silver medal in the 1984 Olympics, who'd died from pancreatic cancer not long before our 25th.

As part of the festivities for our reunion, there were a number of small groups that we could attend to meet classmates who shared our professional and personal interests. There was no shortage of brilliance and accomplishment in my class as witnessed during a cabaret night when the host of NPR's "All Things Considered" greeted the members of the band Semisonic, who'd written the well-known anthem of the decade, "Closing Time." Although they and all the performers were my classmates, I was still struck by the incredible talent that I'd been fortunate enough to be around, and that I now was getting to know over meals, in commencement lines, and on buses that transported us to various events like the Boston Pops, where another famous member of our class performed.

For that reason, I was touched to be asked to appear on a panel devoted to breakthroughs in the areas of science and health that classmates wanted to know about. The moderator was one of the leading medical specialists in eating disorders at a Harvard teaching hospital. The two male panelists with me were well-known for their groundbreaking work in cancer and Alzheimer's treatment. And then there was me.

I listened to my classmates talk about their work in their fields and the research they'd done that had been published in renowned journals. They were impressive and fascinating. As I sat at the front of the room in one of the Science Center classrooms listening to them, I felt a crazy sense of *déjà vu*: the last time I'd sat in this vast auditorium as a miserable bulimic was over 25 years ago and some of the bathrooms where I'd been through purge cycles were only steps from the doors. I certainly hadn't covered myself in glory while at Harvard, where I was supposed to have been at the pinnacle of teen success that was going to make me happy, while the people sharing the stage with me appeared to have been on a different trajectory, one that had included success after success, starting young.

But for some reason, I was sitting with them, about to share my own story, so I told myself that although my path hadn't been so neat up to this point, I still had something important to share. I stood up at the lectern and began to speak.

"Twenty-five years ago, I was not the picture of health and certainly had nothing of value to teach my classmates, but a lot has changed since we graduated, and I'd like to share some of those developments with you because they mirror some of the advances in the fields of addiction and psychology."

Although *My Name is Caroline* had been published fewer than five years after our graduation, I assumed that some people didn't know about it, so I described what the book was about, but quickly brought the audience to the present-day as I talked about my degree from Penn, and the fact that history had been made on Harvard's college campus with Tal's record-breaking class in Positive Psychology. I encouraged everyone to take advantage of the findings of the positive psychology world, and shared some of the work on gratitude, strengths and well-being research, as well as the fact that my next book on goal-setting would be coming out shortly.

By the end of the session, I was proud that I'd proven that I belonged on the panel, especially because I was peppered with questions from the audience about where to go to learn more about positive psychology. Many, it seemed, had fallen into the trap of thinking they'd be happy if they achieved certain heights in life, but were struggling with some of the same issues I'd once felt. When it was over, a number of people lined up to speak to me. At least half of them were classmates who thanked me for writing my first book. They lowered their voices as they shared that they'd battled eating disorders, that my book had helped them decades earlier, and that they wanted to thank me in person for my courage in writing it. Some confided that they still struggled with body image issues and weight, and wanted to know how I'd stayed in recovery for so long.

One of the most surprising conversations was with a male classmate who said that he'd been the producer of a well-known, but controversial, documentary on eating disorders that I had mentioned in my talk as representative of the problems still facing the eating disorder world. The documentary had been featured widely in the media as an honest and searing look at eating disorder treatment, but the message many had taken from it was that full recovery was a rare outcome. Of the four people featured prominently in it, one had died and the others had relapsed and weren't doing well. I had commented that we needed to counter these messages with more uplifting stories of long-term recovery to engender hope that people got better and stayed better. I told him that if I'd seen the documentary in my early twenties, I might have assumed that no one got better, so why bother?

"We never got that feedback," my classmate remarked in surprise as he introduced himself. "We thought we were doing something good!"

I explained that while shining a light on what happened in eating disorder centers and to its patients was important and necessary, it was equally important to devote significant airtime to the fact that people got better and stayed better for a long time, too. Our conversation reminded me of one of the challenges I'd faced in the years after the first book had been published, and a well-known talk show approached me to be a guest on the topic of bulimia. By that time, I'd seen how the focus of these shows still remained on talking about the problem, instead of the solution, so I said I'd come on if I could bring people in recovery with me. I'd been turned down immediately: "I'm sorry. Young and sick makes for better TV."

I was one of the last to leave the Science Center, and I walked slowly out the heavy doors into the fresh air. To my left was Memorial Hall, where I'd visited Harvard's Positive Psychology class two years earlier, and where we were now taking our meals as reunion guests. The sounds of bustling Harvard Square were to the right, where a cacophony of honking, shouting and chanting was audible. Ahead of me were some of the brick and wrought-iron gates ringing the perimeter of the main campus.

I decided to kill some time until I met up with my family again, so I passed through the gates and walked a hundred yards to the iconic statue of John Harvard in the middle of Harvard Yard. How many times had I rushed by this statue as a sad student, going to and from classes, head down, filled with self-doubt, loathing, fear and depression, wishing I could be someone else? I longed to go back and take that young girl into my arms and tell her that everything was going to turn out okay, and that there would be people who would love her unconditionally when she needed them the most, and that she would experience the joy of bearing children and watching them grow up. I wanted to tell her that she'd find fulfillment in school again, ironically while studying happiness, and that she'd also learn how to create that happiness for herself, without food ever being a problem or preoccupation again. I was lost in my thoughts as I just stood there.

I watched tourists pushing their way through the Yard, thronging the statue and taking pictures. It suddenly reminded me of when I'd lined up in the National Cathedral exactly 25 years ago this month, ready to walk down the aisle while tourists took my picture. Some of the most private moments of my life had always been public in one way or another, and now I'd opened my life up to even more scrutiny by sharing so much through my books. Living a private life just wasn't my karma, I smiled to myself, but for some reason, that was the life I was meant to lead, and it was one that I hoped had helped others.

I heard my name being called and saw Haywood and the three children coming my way, fresh from their own activities. I watched thoughtfully as my husband, whom I'd met here at Harvard, and the three biggest joys of my life, approach me. It was hard not to contrast the Caroline of 1983 with the Caroline who was standing here now. I'd come back to Harvard to celebrate my reunion, but had instead come back to realize that Harvard hadn't been wasted at all, and that it had actually been the crucible for all of the good that had later occurred in my life. I'd met my husband here, but I'd also learned the lesson that the happiness I'd thought Harvard would bring didn't exist, and that I'd have to find a new way to live and approach life if I were ever to feel healthy or contented. Today, standing here in the Yard, I knew that feeling, and I had Harvard to thank for launching me into orbit, and then bringing me back to share my findings—which were just as relevant to health as the findings on cancer and Alzheimer's disease that I'd heard today.

I knew in that moment that I had nothing left to heal from my eating disorder, and that every facet of my life that had been disrupted by the bulimia had now been faced and resolved for good. The hobbies were back, my body was healed, my family demons had been dealt with, and I had gone back to school at a time and in a way that had changed my life. I'd once thought that simply stopping the purging had been the triumph, but now I knew that many other things had had to be dealt with in order for this deep-rooted issue to finally reach its conclusion.

I'd come full circle and I was a better person for everything I'd gone through. My future looked bright. Life was good.

"Let's go pack up," I said. "It's time to go home. We've done everything we need to do here."

I walked away from the John Harvard statue with satisfaction. My decades of healing myself were finally concluded.

248

# EPILOGUE

A lot has happened in the years since I graduated from Penn and attended my 25th reunion at Harvard, and while not everything has been rosy all the time, life has continued to be very good, for which I am grateful.

A few developments will help tie up loose ends from the story I've told here, while also illuminating what I set out to give to others by writing this book. I want to reiterate that I didn't write *Positively Caroline* to put myself forward as someone who wants to tell others how to live, what to do, or to glamorize myself in any way. I was so reluctant to write this book at times that it has taken me longer to start and finish it than it has taken me to write my other five books.

But I kept returning to one key point that compelled me to finally finish it: I got into recovery as a young adult and stayed in recovery throughout the next several decades without relapsing or becoming addicted to anything else, while morphing into the healthiest and happiest version of myself. This type of outcome is something we need to hear about and see more of in the media so that it becomes a normal and expected fact for people with eating disorders—much like what we have seen with role models like Betty Ford, Dick Van Dyke and Eric Clapton in the field of alcoholism and drug addiction.

Many other people could have written this book, as there are people with as much recovery as me who have valuable stories to tell, but the platform I created in 1988 with *My Name is Caroline* opened me up to decades of questions about what had happened to me later. I hope this story will do as much good as the first book, but in a different way.

The book I began as part of my Capstone project at Penn became *Creating Your Best Life* and was published by Sterling Publishing in early 2009. It has been translated into multiple languages, with sold-out editions of both hardback and paperback, and it is even used in educational settings as a textbook because of its rigorous scientific approach to the subject. As I had hoped, it was the first popular book on goal accomplishment that showed where the science of success intersects with the science of well-being, giving the public an alternative to the anecdotal and slick goal books that once predominated in the market. I was especially gratified that the esteemed Library Journal awarded it a coveted red star review in February 2009, noting that it was "one of the best books of its kind."

Haywood and I, who are approaching our 30th anniversary, remain in love and committed to each other, and despite literally growing up together, we've managed to dodge and roll with every new challenge that has faced us. It hasn't been easy, with some times harder than others, but a foundation of mutual respect, laughter, and the decision to wake up every day and do whatever needs to be done together has served us well. I'm grateful that he has always believed in me and my abilities, and that when he took a chance on asking out a lonely bulimic in a pair of baggy overalls in 1981, he paved the way for me to feel the unconditional acceptance and love that allowed me to seek help a few years later when I hit my last bottom.

Our children have grown up and continue to bring us tremendous joy, as well as the requisite heartbreak that comes with watching them fall down and figure out how to get back up without us doing it for them. Haywood IV graduated from the University of Cincinnati in 2012, where he captained the swim team and got an accounting degree, and he now works in an accounting firm in Northern Virginia. Most important, when his swimming career almost ended against his will during two tumultuous years at the University of Maryland, I told him about the "peak-end" rule I'd learned at Penn and encouraged him to make sure that he ended his swim career in a way that would always bring him pride and satisfaction. He did just that, which turned out to be one of the toughest and best decisions of his life. It took guts not to quit his beloved sport completely, as well as hard work to start all over at a different school. But the friendships and life experiences he gained by transferring to Cincinnati, thanks to the gracious welcome of swim coach Monty Hopkins, are character investments that will pay rich dividends for the rest of his life.

Samantha is a rower and American History enthusiast at Brown University, and she is just as exuberant and talkative a young woman as she was as a young girl, who knows what she wants and goes after it with dogged determination and grit. In her late teens she faced some dissatisfaction with her body, and careened around the scale a bit before finding a steady and happy place that doesn't result in obsessive behaviors or self-destructive eating habits. When I found out I was pregnant with a "big girl," I set the goal of doing my best to raise a young woman who had the courage to be herself, regardless of what society wanted her to look like, and I think she has succeeded in becoming that person.

Bayard is near the end of his senior year in high school and still finds solace and happiness in reading and learning as many facts as he can, which landed him the honor of becoming captain of his high school's "It's Academic" team in 11th grade. He is also one of the 120 students to win the prestigious Presidential Scholar award in 2013 for academic merit—the nation's top honor for high school seniors. His favorite sport, football, was taken away by a career-ending hit that led to major shoulder surgery in eleventh grade, precipitating a tough readjustment to his goals. Just like his siblings, though, it was adversity that caused Bayard's character strengths to emerge, and the way he has dealt with the challenges of the last year has been more impressive to me than any of the intellectual successes he's achieved in life that came more easily to him.

My recovery continues to be strong, but since I recently entered my fifties, I'm experiencing a new stage of body changes and emotional shifts that come with having a mostly empty nest and increasing hormonal upheavals. The media reports on midlife eating disorders point to some of what I'm facing as common triggers for relapse, or even the onset of an eating disorder, but I think I'm on solid ground when it comes to predicting that I'll be okay; I've done enough footwork and created enough resilience to weather the difficulties that come my way.

In writing this book over the last five years, I've sifted through every possible aspect of my behavior and thinking that might be helpful to others who are trying to get into eating disorder recovery and stay there. Through my stories, which pick up where my first book left off, I hope I've given readers who are looking for long-term recovery, or just authentic happiness that is independent of external achievements, some ideas about what they might want to add to their lives, or some new thoughts about how they can challenge some of their existing beliefs or behaviors.

Here are some of the factors I believe have played the most important role in getting me safely to midlife without relapse:

- I stopped drinking alcohol within the first year of my recovery from bulimia. I had all of the genetic seeds and behaviors typical of emergent alcoholics, and I decided that my life would be better if I never altered my mood in that way again. I also heard in self-help meetings how common it was to switch addictions, and I wanted to try to avoid that at all costs because I knew that my own personal food abstinence would be shaky if I lived that way. Later at Penn, I learned that alcohol is the one proven deterrent to maintaining willpower in the face of temptation, so by being sober, I avoided hundreds of situations where I'm sure I would have been vulnerable to faulty, self-destructive thinking and behavior.

- I held fast to the habits and thinking created in early recovery that were often elegant in their simplicity, yet very effective. These included always having at least three balanced meals each day, avoiding tempting situations where food would be unlimited, stopping at one helping regardless of the food, and remembering always that "the first bite" would always be "the best," so why overdo it, anyway? The slogans I saw on walls and heard frequently continue to resonate in my head and make sense—First Things First. Let Go and Let God. One Day at a Time. If You Pray Why Worry, and If You Worry, Why Pray? Easy Does It. Have An Attitude of Gratitude.

- I finally learned that I had inherited a genetic legacy of addiction, depression and ADHD, and I started on a regimen of medications that I continue to this day. In early recovery, I believed that my success was all about effort and proper attitude, but it wasn't until these other areas were stable that I realized how underlying issues had probably contributed to my eating disorder, and that they too needed to be addressed.

- I haven't voluntarily weighed myself since 1984, nor have I ever owned a scale in adulthood. Some people prefer to monitor their weight as part of their recovery, but for me, this is a loaded proposition. My doctors know what I weigh, and they have all promised to tell me if something changes or they have concerns about me, and that has removed any unnecessary emotional stress I might have about this topic. My clothes fit from year to year, and without doing anything extreme to maintain my figure, I continue to be the same size, year in and year out, without drama, diets or any type of obsessive approaches to my life.

- I did something that was very hard, and also very controversial among some people: I eventually had to cut off all contact with my mother because she finally crossed a line with me that was unforgivable. She still lives within two blocks of my home but has rarely acknowledged my presence, or my children's presence, in years. Those who don't understand people with borderline personality disorder (BPD) have given me misguided and hurtful advice around how to handle her behavior, assuming that I'm simply an unforgiving person. But I'm very indebted to a series of books that were published in the mid 1990's about the specific challenges faced by children of borderline parents. After meeting dozens of women like me who have been tormented by a mother for most of their lives, I saw a pattern that I wanted to write about. One of the most helpful books I read discussed how borderline mothers often select one child to despise and they try to "steal that child's soul" and destroy all of their joy. Eating disorders are very common among these children, and it's no accident that I fit right into this mold. There is no pain like knowing that your mother has no interest in you or love for you, and that you'll never know what it's like to be missed or cherished by the person who gave birth to you. But that is the hand that I was dealt, and for my own well-being, as well as my own children's—who often returned from visiting her with stories about how they had to hear me openly criticized and derided—I made the decision in 2005 that I had to create concrete boundaries around seeing or talking to her that others might find cruel or unfeeling. I don't recommend this step for everyone because it is one of the most emotionally wrenching things you can do to protect yourself, but it was the right one for me and many professionals were helpful with this decision. I thought long and hard about revealing this facet of my adult life and ongoing growth in this book, but I ultimately decided that any book designed to help people deal with the emotional roadblocks that come up in maintaining long-term recovery would be inauthentic if I chose to whitewash or ignore something that has been so significant in my life, and that I have found is so common among eating disordered women like myself.

- On a similar note, I kept pushing through the issues that came up within my family by seeking the right help and creating a "family" around me of carefully-chosen individuals who never shirked from telling me what I needed to hear and who supported me in hard times. This included my godmother Pat, my coach Judy Feld, my therapist Shep, my female friends, and other "wise" elders who were constant and kind presences in my life and in my children's lives. At Penn, the lesson that "other people matter" was hammered home so often as part of the recipe for a fulfilling life that I have made even more efforts in recent years to spend time with people who not only make me a better person, but whose lives I hope I enrich, as well. One note from the research: women need at least three good friends, and it's better to go deep with those people instead of superficial and wide, so I am thoughtful about who I allow into my world, and I advise all of my clients that it "ought to be hard" to make your "A" team of friends because of their potential impact on you.

- Building on this point: I try to be around positive situations and positive people whenever possible. In early recovery, I was told to "stick with the winners," which boiled down to being around people with strong recovery programs who could serve as role models. At Penn, I learned about social contagion theory and how different behaviors from quitting smoking to becoming obese are contagious, and it explained to me why I naturally thrived in upbeat settings, and how that might have contributed to keeping my recovery intact. Again, since learning this research, I've made even more of an effort to be cognizant of who brings out the best in me, and whose behavior I want to "catch" whenever I'm pursuing my own goals.

- I stumbled into a very healing set of behaviors that gave me closure on many of the areas that had been discussed in therapy, but never completely healed. As I recounted in this book, I was frequently hit by both my father and mother when I was growing up and right up until the night before I got married, but pursuing a black belt in Hapkido taught me how to spar aggressively and fairly with others. Talking about the abuse in therapy had been helpful in some ways, but I was unexpectedly empowered by stepping into the sparring ring in a protected way. Although I didn't go into the martial arts for this benefit, there's no question that I unwittingly found a way to get at some lingering inner demons. Similarly, I had lost both swimming and piano to my bulimic behavior, and when I went back as an adult to voluntarily pursue these activities for the sheer joy they gave me, I once again found that some unexpected healing occurred. No therapist had ever once suggested that I return to activities that had ended in unhealthy ways, but when I did this, I found that all of the talking and writing about those losses didn't touch the power of doing that activity again of my own volition. Again, it was Penn where I got the language to understand why this was so important: the "peak-end" rule dictated that how something ends is how you remember it, so returning to these lost behaviors gave me the power to "end" them in positive ways, giving me a profound feeling of peace and completion. Going back to school was another demonstration of how this approach worked for me; Harvard was a bulimic nightmare, but at Penn, I got a second chance to be the student I was capable of being, thus healing that wound.

- Disentangling what I wanted to accomplish versus what others expected me to accomplish was an important piece of figuring out where to set my sights going forward. In *My Name is Caroline*, my sole purpose was to get into recovery, and I did. But when the book ended, I had no other defined direction, so I had to learn a lot more about who I was and where I wanted to go in life in order to stay in recovery. This meant that I had to repeatedly try and fail at a variety of endeavors while continuing to pick myself up and keep going. At Penn, I learned that I'd been governed for most of my life by pursuing extrinsic goals, which were not conducive to wellbeing because they didn't reflect my own values and desires. As my adult life unfolded, I became clearer about this, and my passion for understanding the difference between these types of goals led me to become a coach with a specialty in working with others to identify and pursue the ambitions that would bring them the greatest fulfillment and wellbeing. If I hadn't developed myself past my earliest definitions of success and challenged myself to live a regret-free life, my unhappiness could have eventually overwhelmed my recovery.

- I continue to seek novelty and challenge, regardless of where it might be, because it keeps me fresh, happy and learning. At Penn, I learned that one of my top strengths is zest, and I realize that when I lead with this trait of "*joie de vivre*," I am not only at my best, I am happier, too. Research has also found that the brain loves novelty, so I have sought to include new sports challenges, educational challenges and professional challenges that are out of my comfort zone so that I never get stale.

I deepened my spiritual faith by joining Community Bible Study during my year at Penn. Jon Haidt, a University of Virginia professor, researcher and author told us at the end of his teaching weekend that "the happiest people have spiritual role models," and that's all it took for me to call a friend, Terry Harris, who took me to my first meeting, where I've found a lot of new friends, learning, and a greater peace.

As I enter the second half of my life, I feel ready for a whole new set of adventures that will physically, emotionally and spiritually challenge me. I have knocked a number of goals off my bucket list, but I have a lot more waiting for me. I doubt I'll ever feel the need to write another auto-biographical book, so I want to close this one with profound gratitude for the people who have given me the gift of their love, time and guidance over several decades, and I hope that many other people will discover, as I did, that it was only by having cracks in my life that the sun was allowed to shine through and make me blossom.

# ACKNOWLEDGEMENTS

This book took me more than five years, from start to finish, to complete, so there are multiple people to thank. Without them, I wouldn't have the insights to heal or the time to write this story.

My husband, Haywood, and my three children, Haywood IV, Samantha and Bayard didn't just read drafts over the years, they allowed me to tell their stories too. Having a mother or wife who is a writer can be a liability, particularly when it comes to memoirs, and they couldn't have been more supportive. I'm fortunate also to have a brother and sister, Bill and Liz Adams, who are generous in every possible way and didn't ask me to change a word.

My agent, Ivor Whitson, and his wife Ronnie, are a major reason why this book is being published. They rolled with the early punches as another book contract interfered with writing this book, and also backed me in deciding that certain themes in this book were too important to leave out. Their support gave me the editorial freedom to tell an honest story. Through Ivor, I met Ann LaFarge, whose storied career in publishing was put to good use as she line-edited my book in the old-fashioned way: with paper and pencil. I am lucky she was assigned to me.

I have created a core group of people who have played, and continue to play, meaningful roles that gave me the courage to heal and come forward, and who also simply keep me organized. My godmother, Pat Griffith, has been the mother and mentor I needed, and Marc Hafkin was another voice of reason and calm in turbulent times. Judy Feld was the first person to believe in my coaching abilities and still guides me in my professional life.

I am also fortunate to be surrounded by a team of people who have become close friends, and who have given me confidence in their areas of expertise: Tasha Bates styles everything I wear, Soroor Mohammed pushes me to change my hair and take risks when I don't want to, Paul Thomas has been my weight-lifting and martial arts guru for fifteen years, and Ellen

Levanda has brought her Ukranian beauty secrets to me and the entire Washington D.C. area. Scott Robinson has created pictures, headshots and videos at the drop of a hat, and my webhost and web designer, Debbie Mahony, has been behind every overhaul of my "brand" for many years, including designing this book's cover and helping me to get this story onto the internet in a variety of cutting-edge ways. Ruth Benavides allowed me to occupy a Denny's booth for hours on multiple occasions when I had nowhere else to write, and I'm fortunate that she continues to be a support system in my life.

My mastermind group of female support listened to me agonize about finishing this book for years, but they never stopped believing in me and this story. Thank you Victoria Aronoff, Mrim Boutla, Karen Collias, Denise Harrington, Holly Mak, Andrea McCarren, Katherine McGreivey and Nancy Mitchell. Every woman should have the good fortune to benefit from the type of brainstorming, laughter and love I experience at our monthly meetings.

The story of Renewal, the company my husband and I formed to create a freestanding residential center for eating disorder recovery, plays a large role in the early pages of this book, and there are people who supported that work and who should be publicly acknowledged. They include Dr. Al Powell, Joann Blackman, Chipper Hoff and the Morgan-Keller construction company. My husband and I also are grateful for the support of family members and friends who donated the seed money that unfortunately never blossomed into the investment we had hoped for—you know who you are and your support and love throughout the long process often kept us going. We've said thank you before on multiple occasions, but there will never be enough expressions of gratitude for that early support, particularly as Renewal fell apart and we couldn't repay any of the money.

Positive Psychology taught me to value relationships as the greatest of gifts, and I hope everyone knows how much they've meant to me. If I haven't said it enough, I'll say it again: Thank you all.

CAROLINE ADAMS MILLER

49532474R00156

Made in the USA
Middletown, DE
19 October 2017